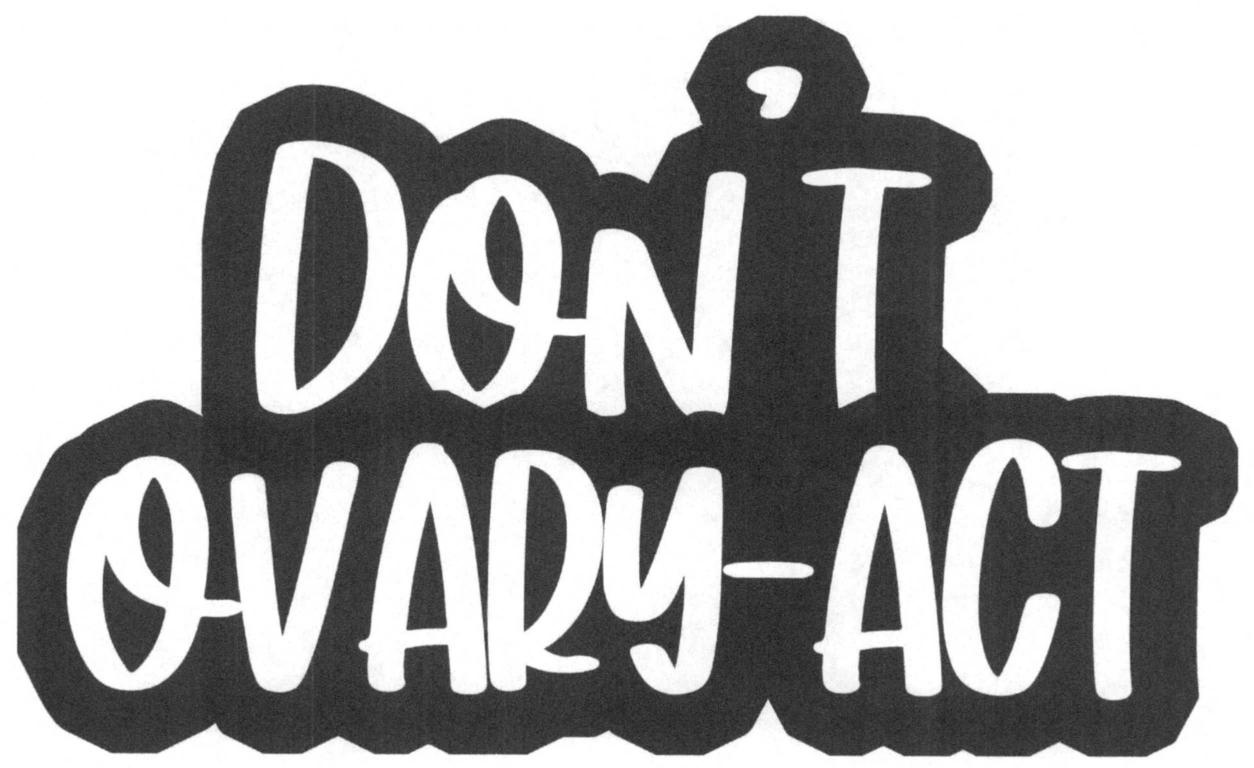

Copyright © 2020 by Buzzle Press

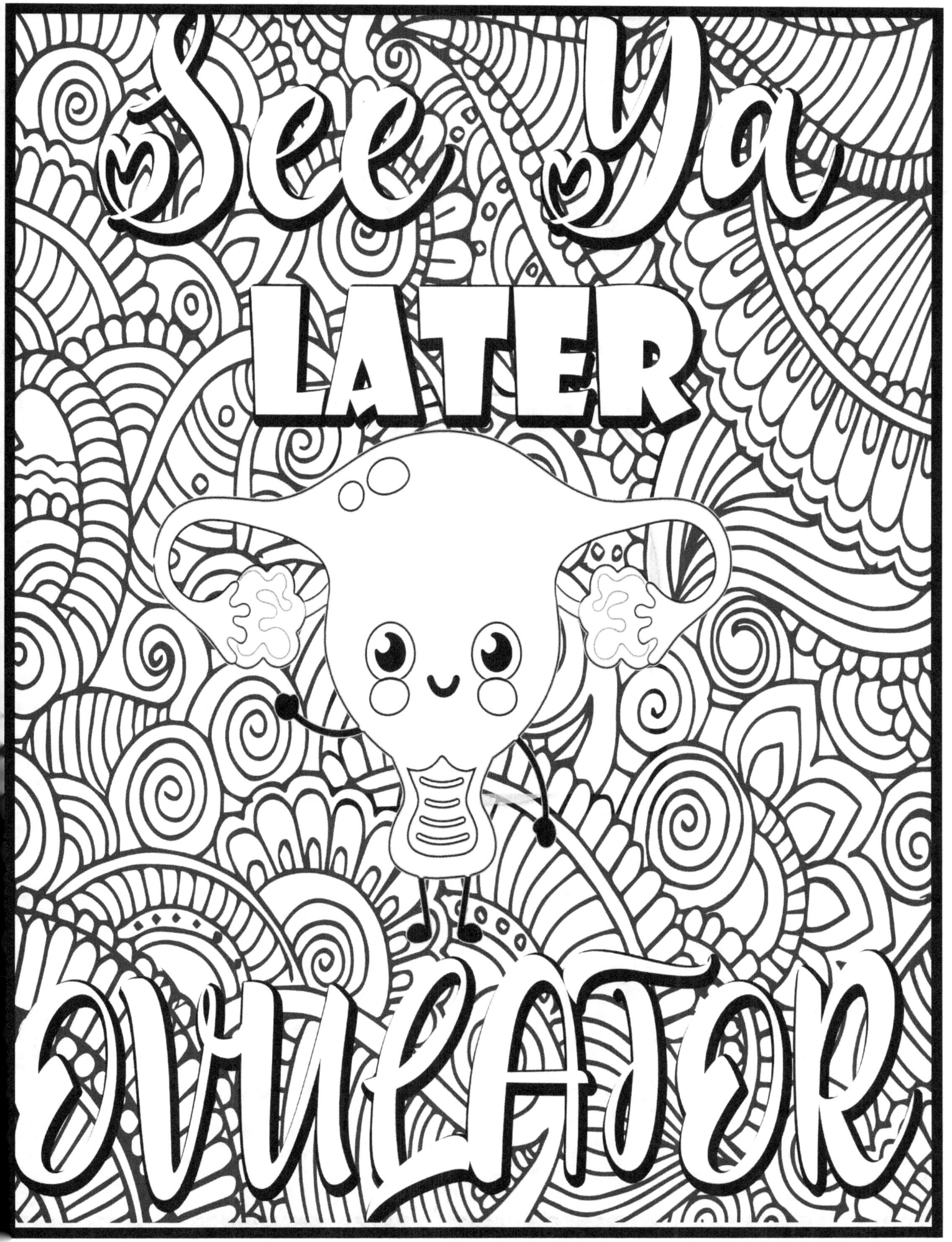

See Ya
LATER
OVULATOR

SUPER COOL HYSTERECTOMY SURVIVOR

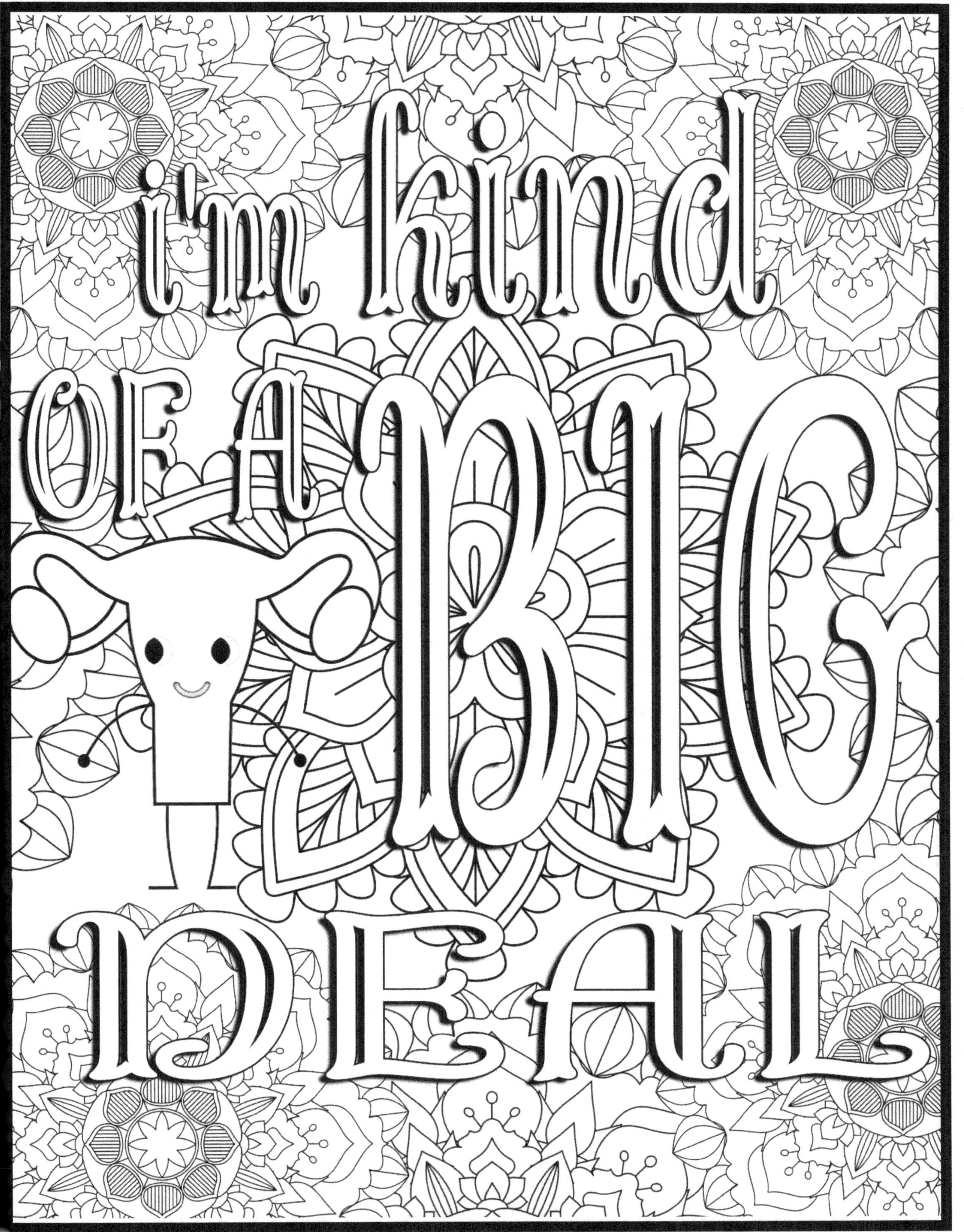

i'm kind
of a
BIG
DEAL

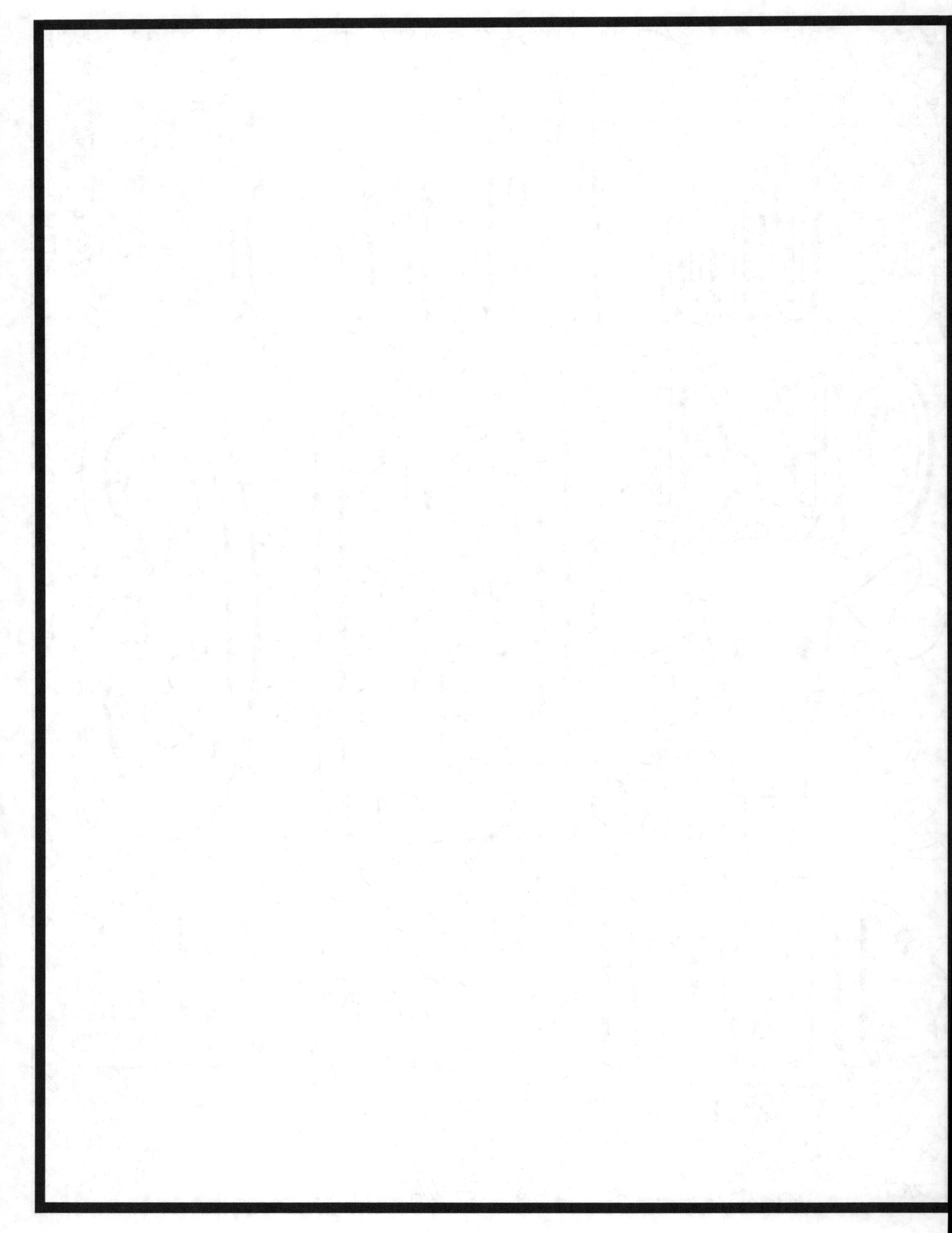

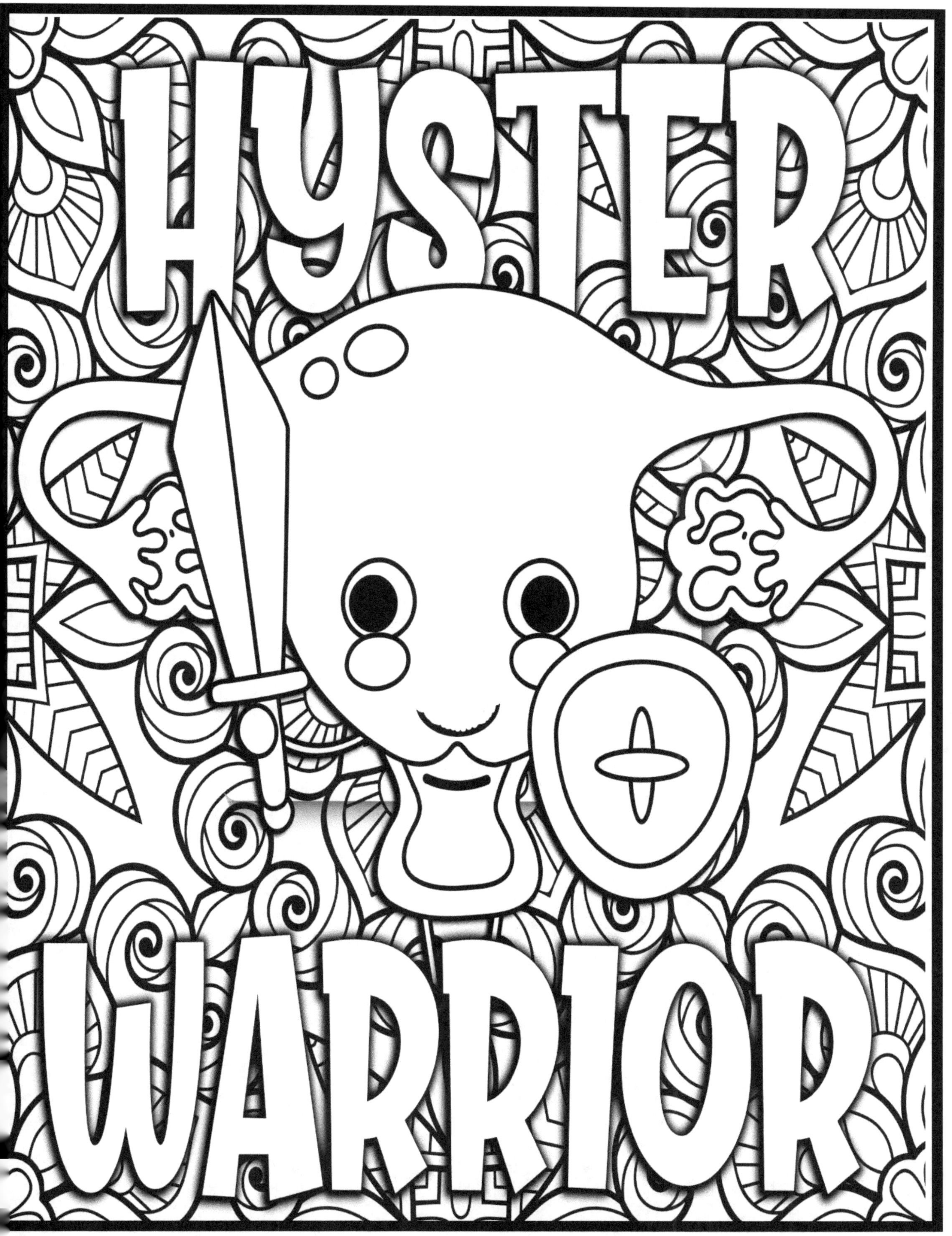

HYSTER
WARRIOR

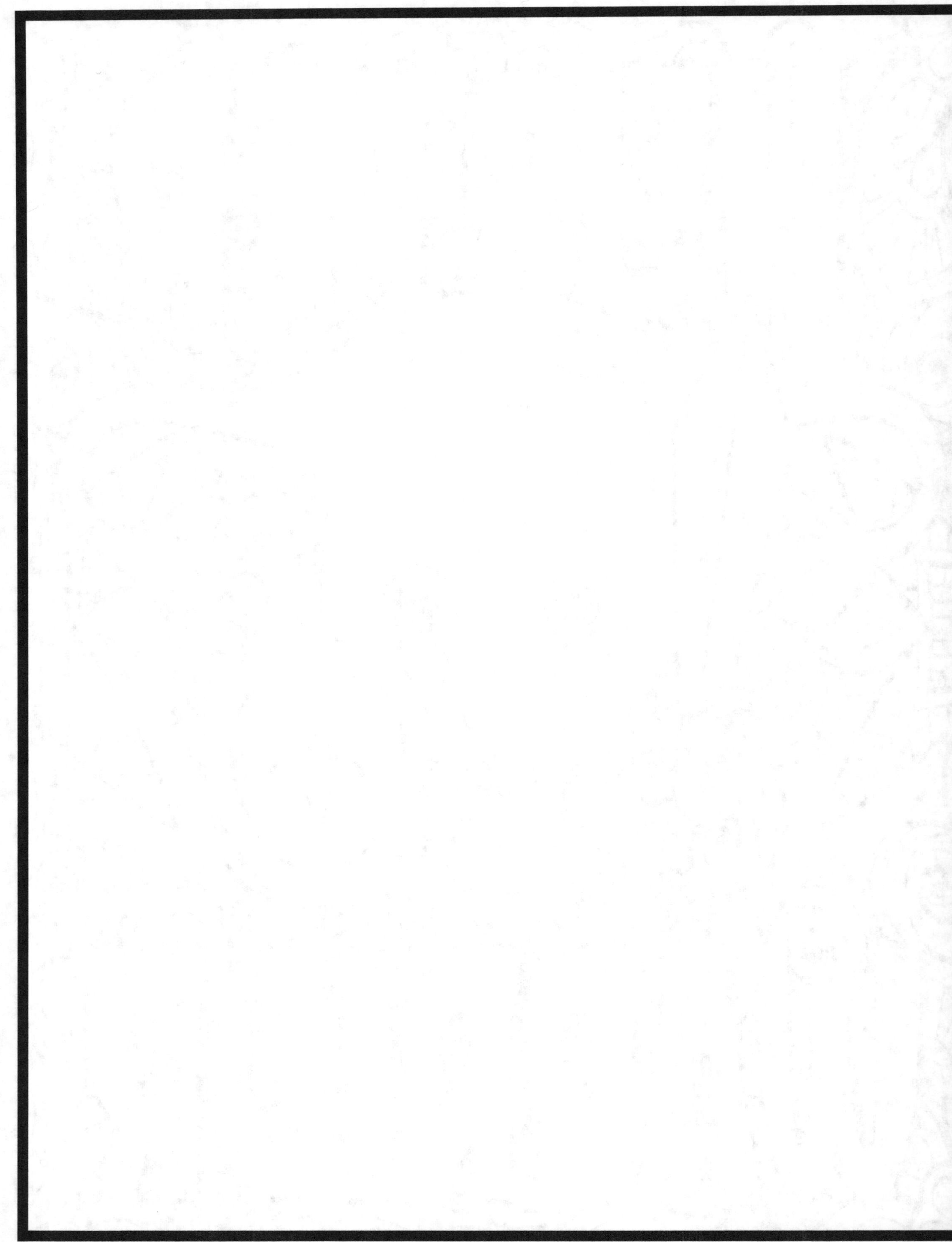

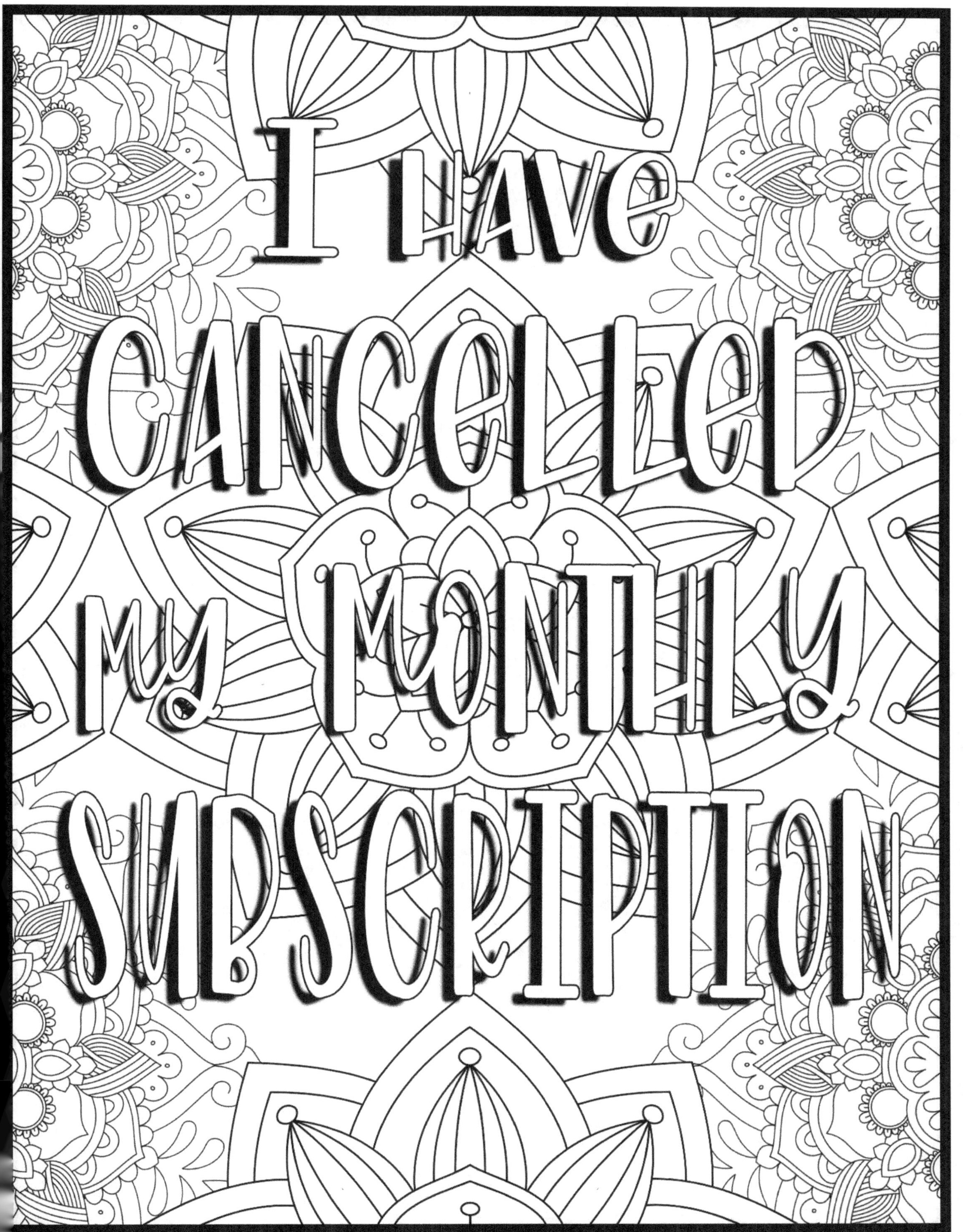
I HAVE CANCELLED MY MONTHLY SUBSCRIPTION

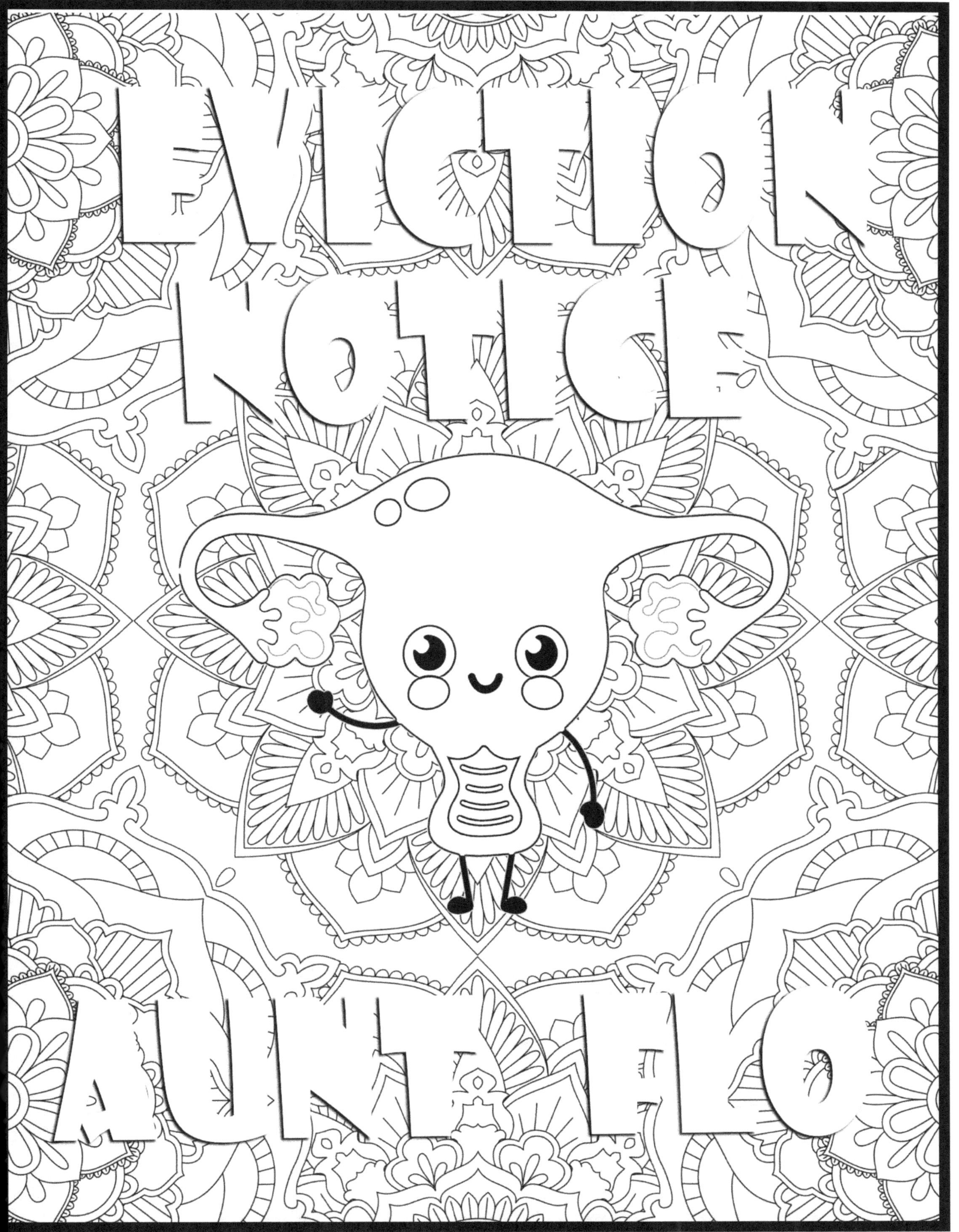

EVICTION
NOTICE
AUNT FLO

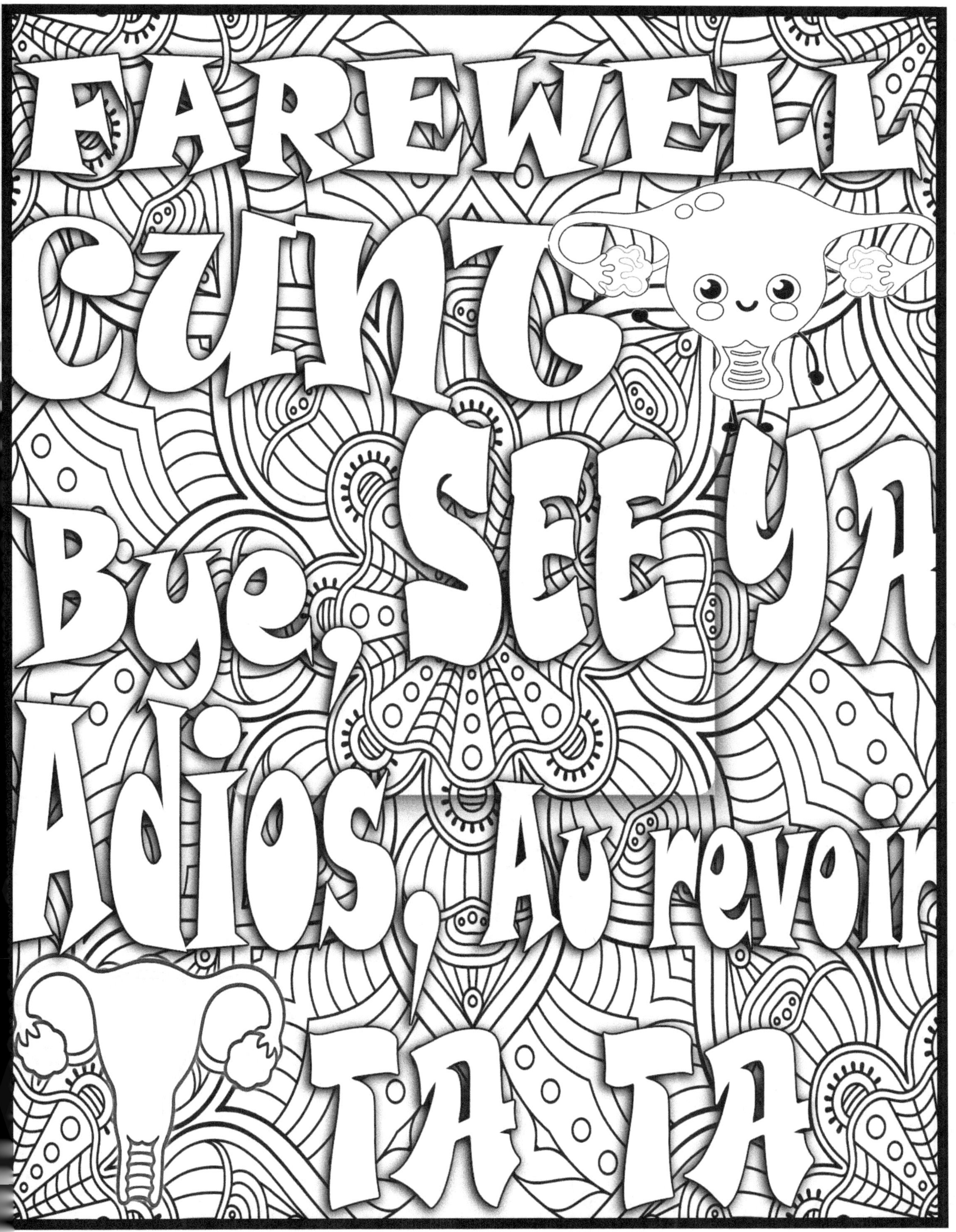

FAREWELL
CUNT
BYE, SEE YA
ADIOS, Au revoir
TA TA

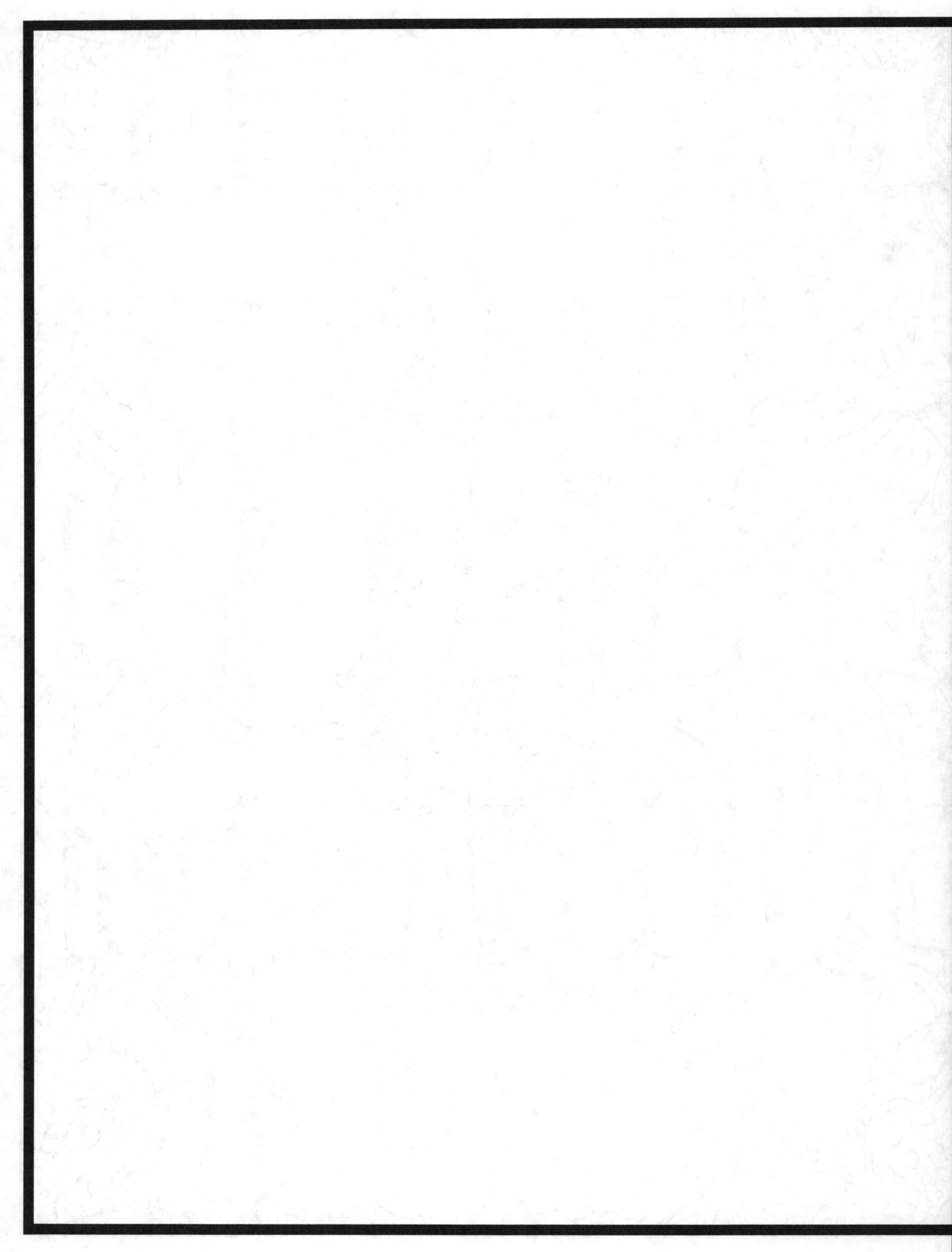

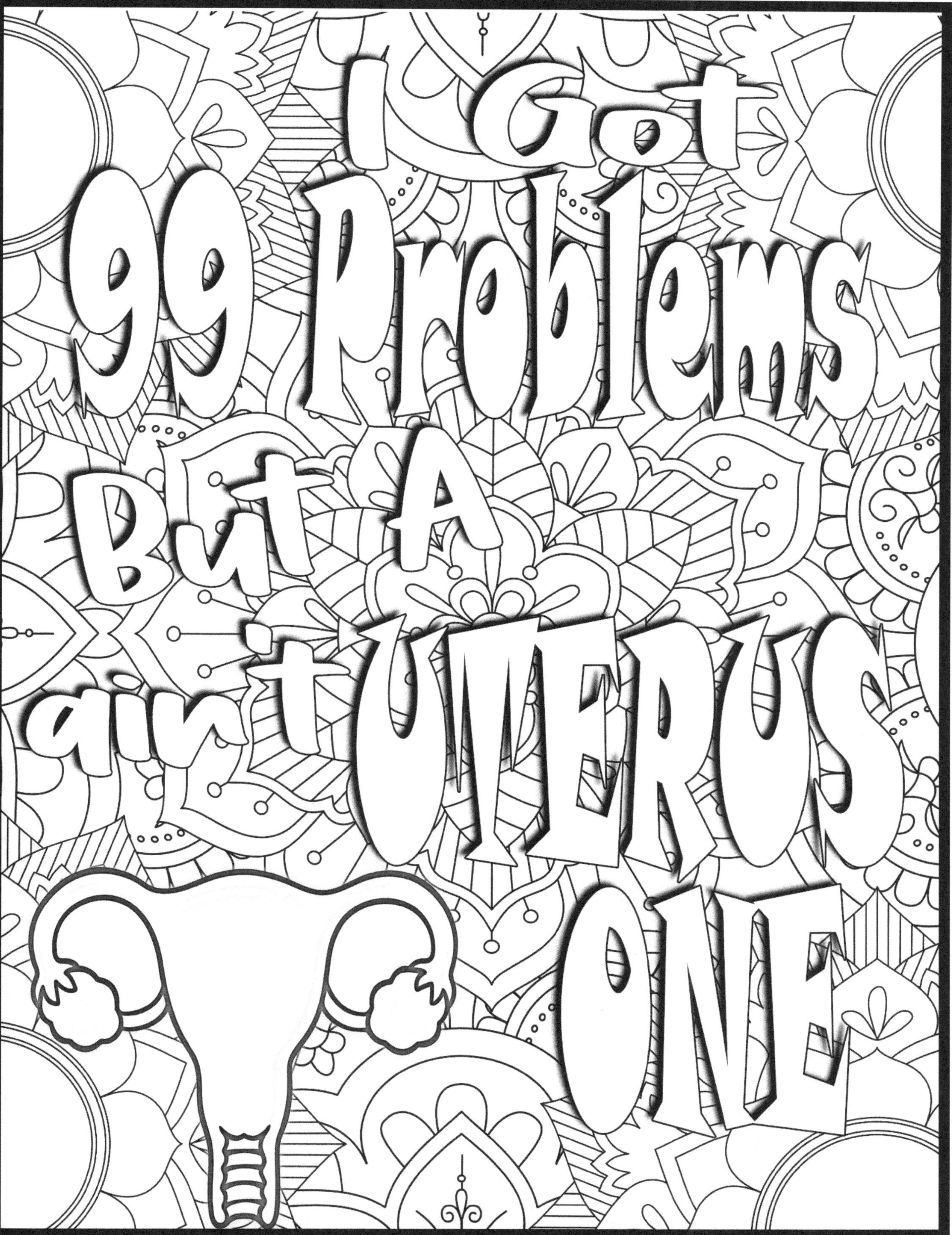

I Got
99 Problems
But A
ain't UTERUS
ONE

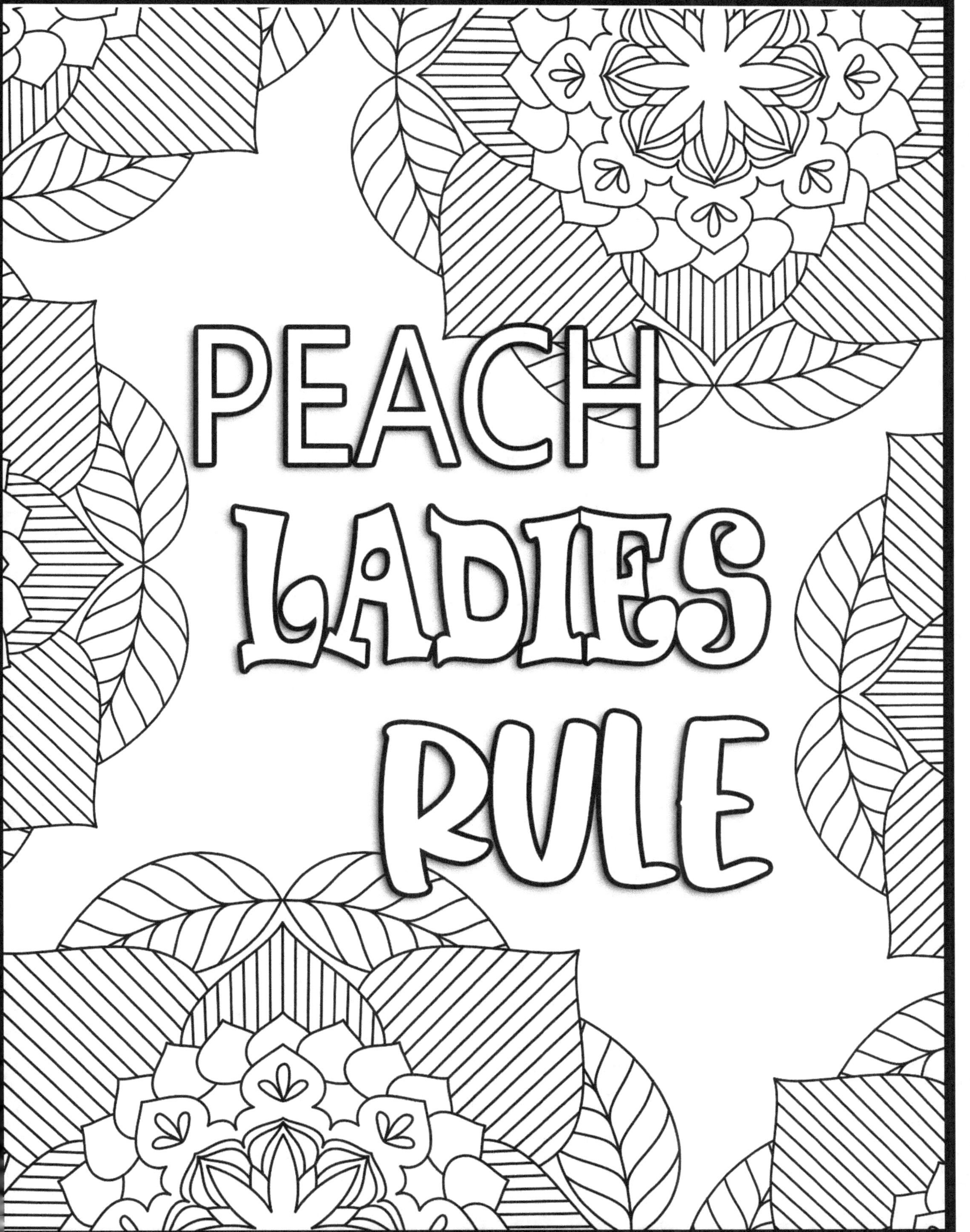

PEACH
LADIES
RULE

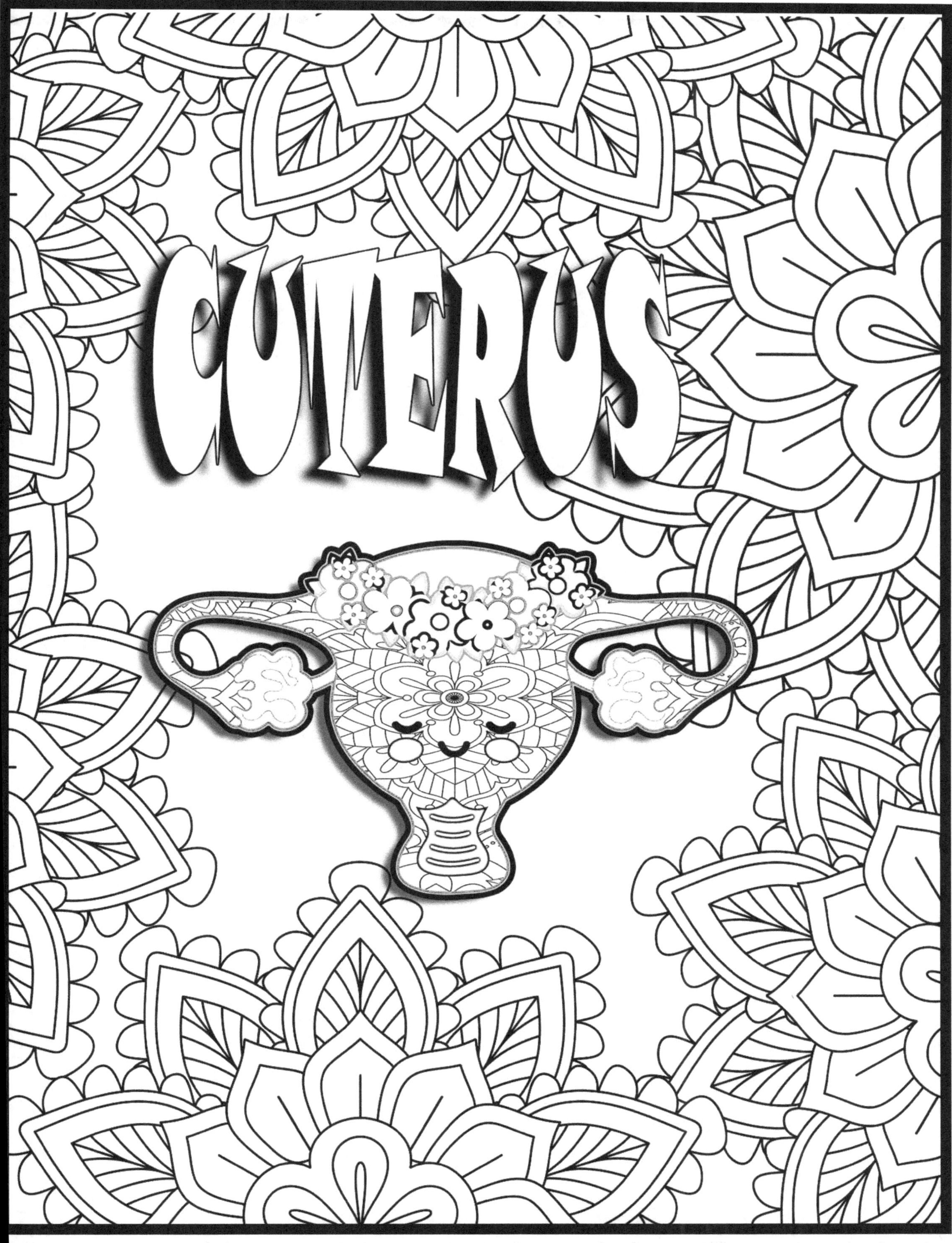
CUTERUS

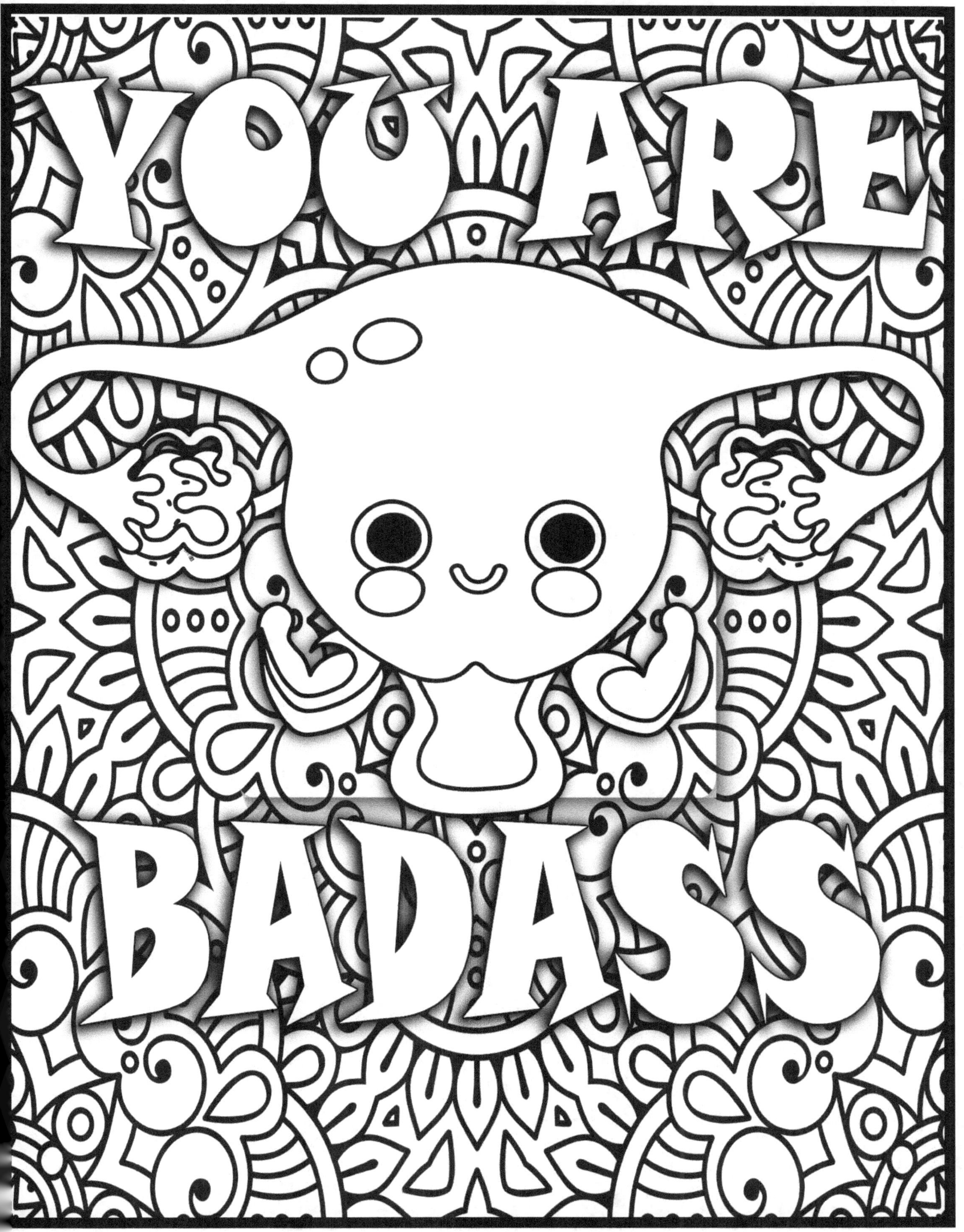

YOU ARE
BADASS

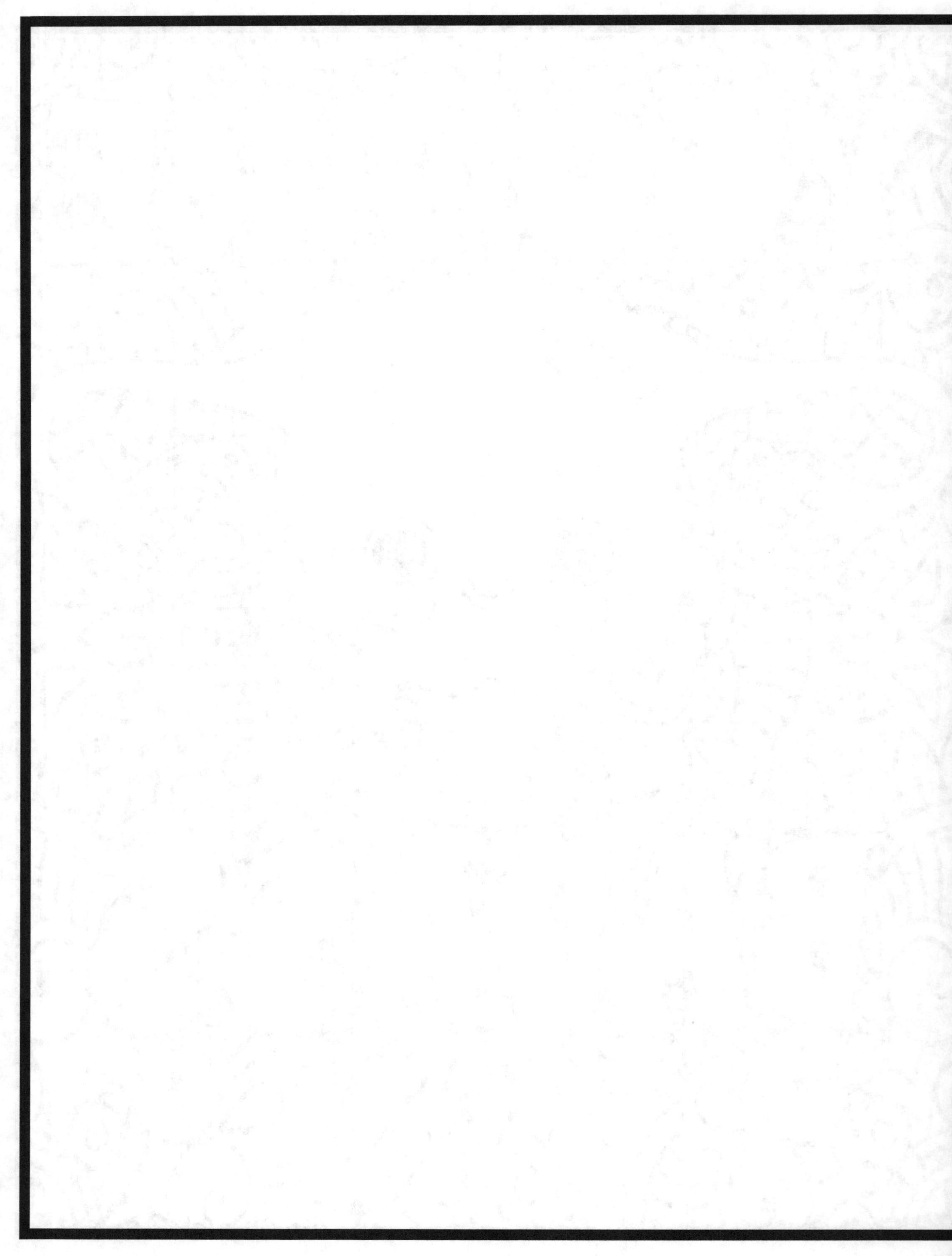

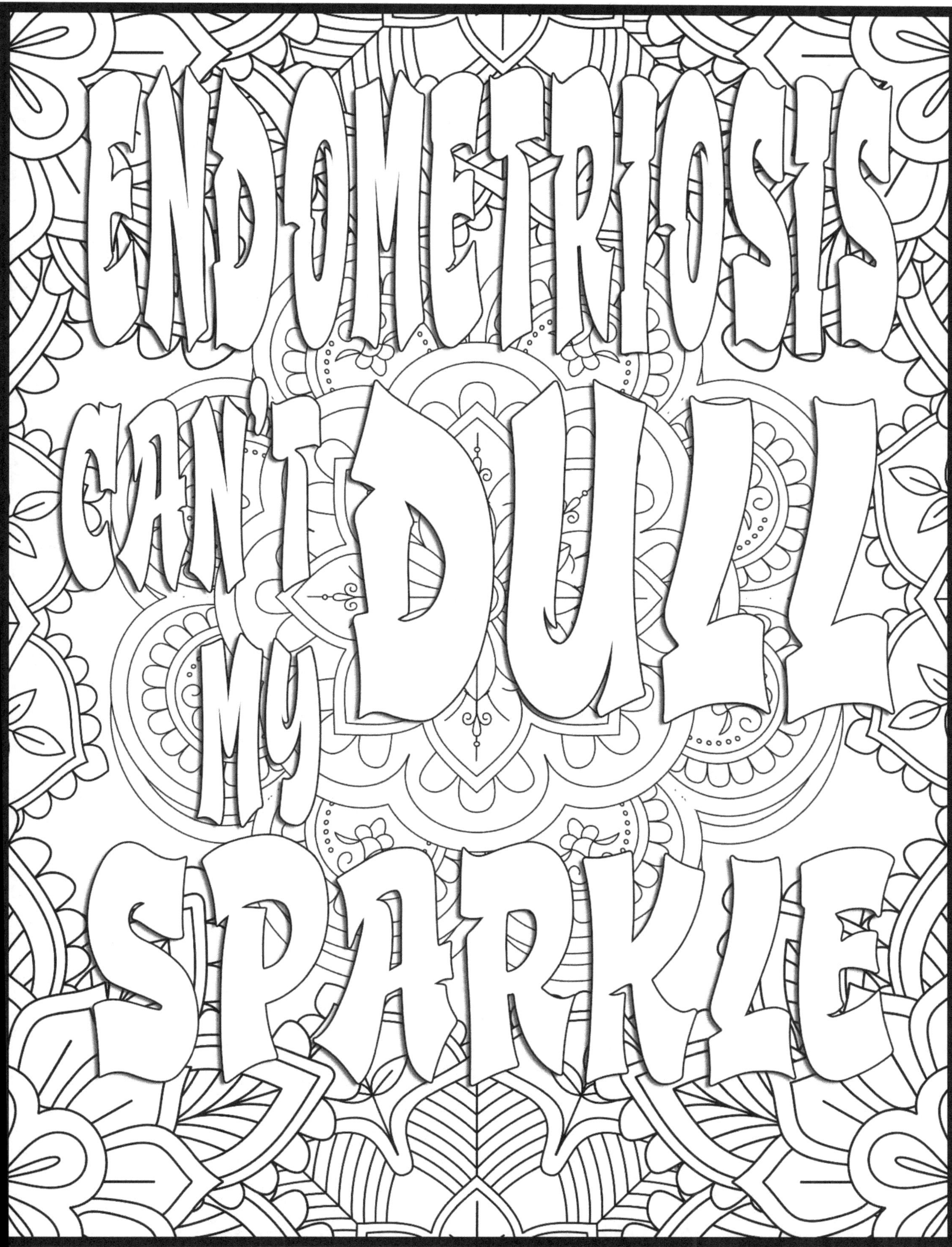

ENDOMETRIOSIS
CAN'T DULL MY
SPARKLE

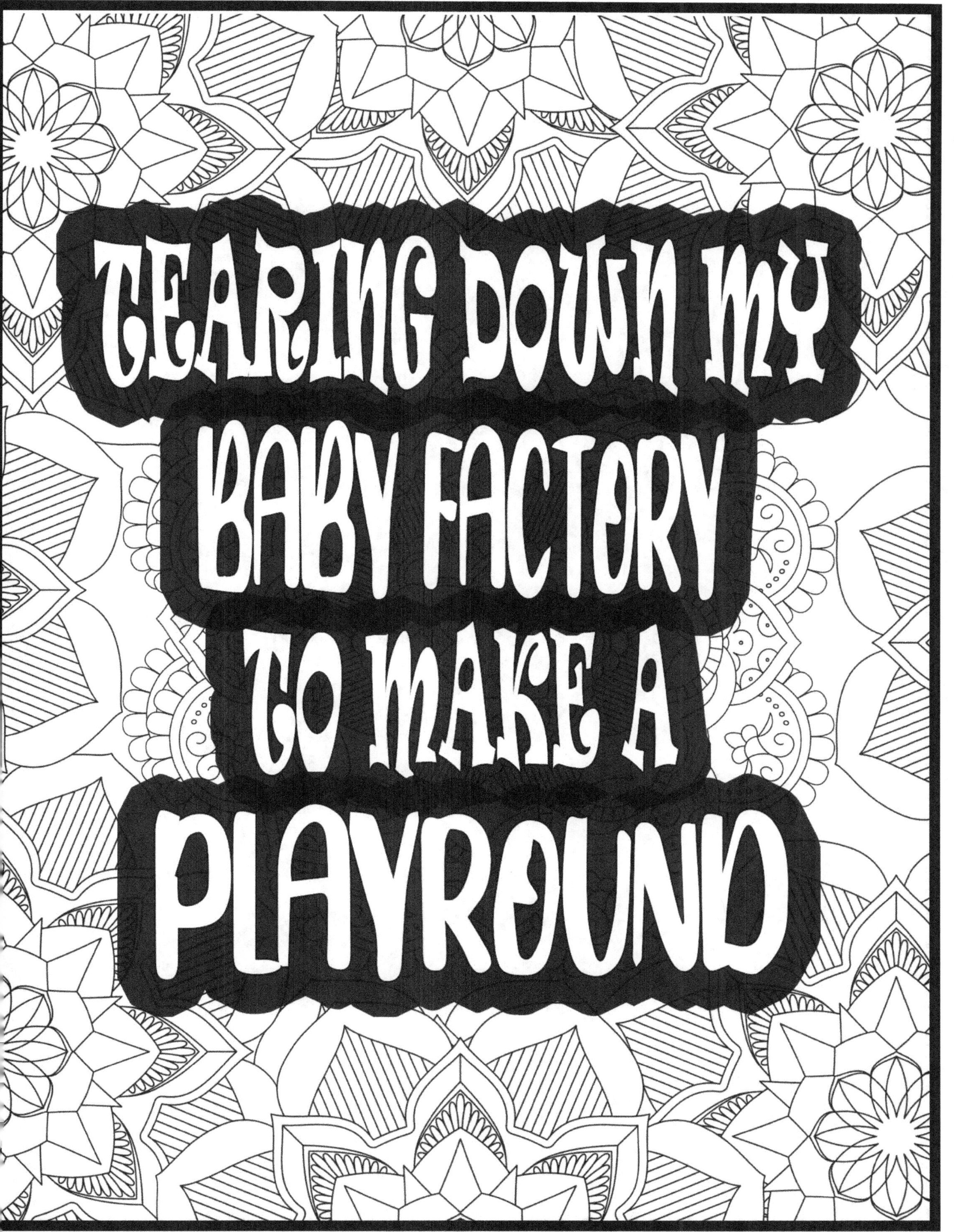
TEARING DOWN MY
BABY FACTORY
TO MAKE A
PLAYROUND

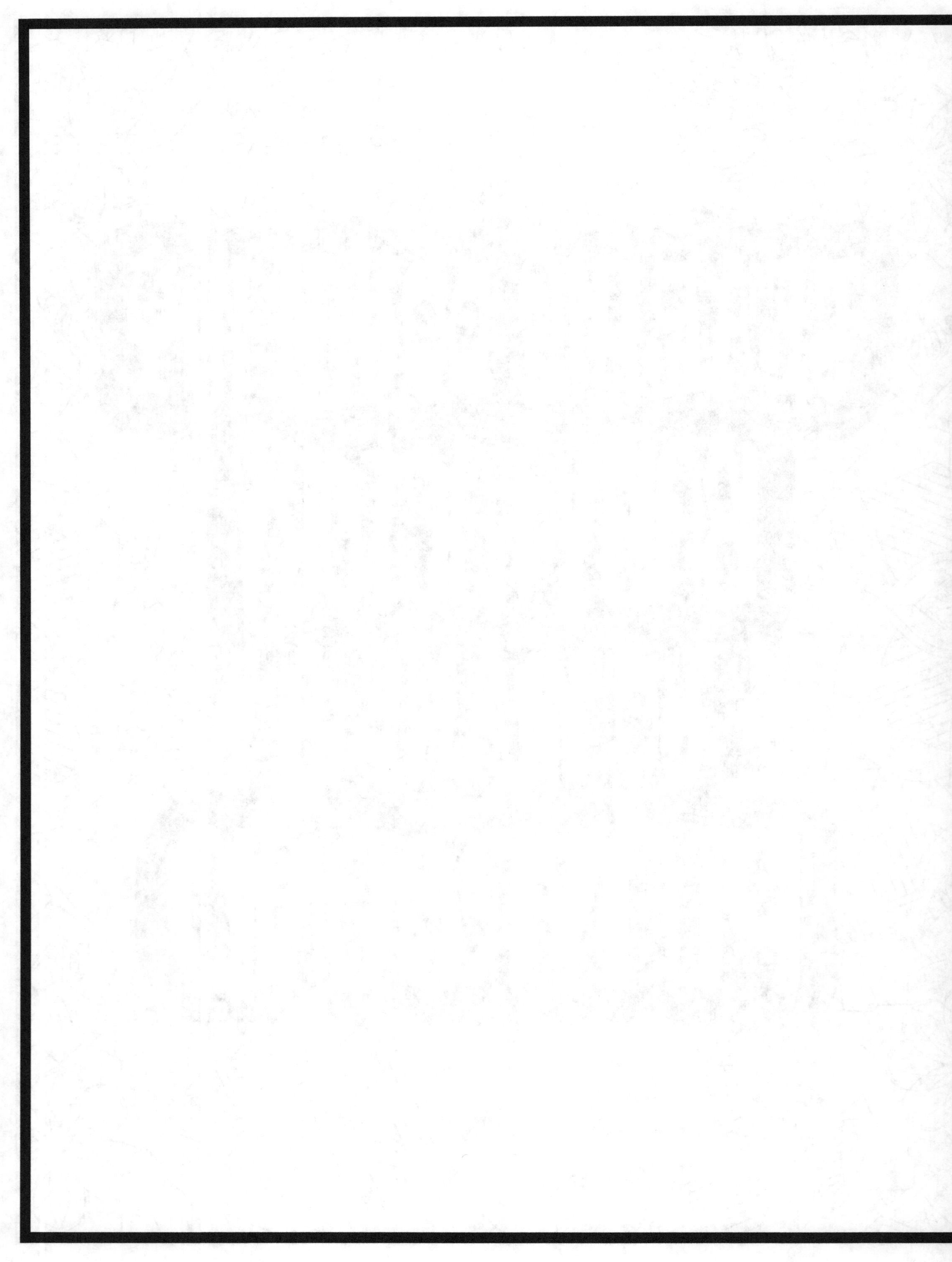

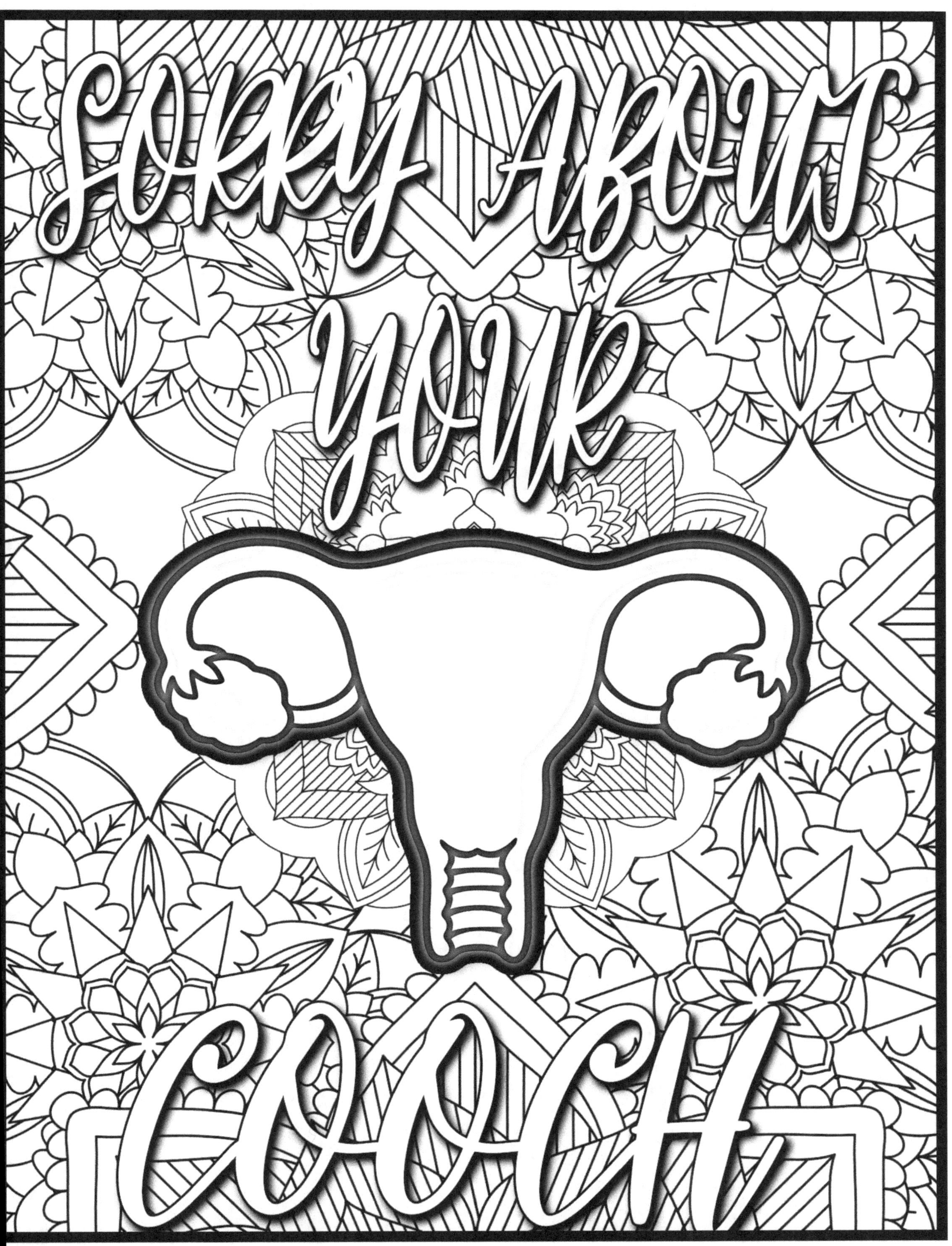

SORRY ABOUT
YOUR
COOCH

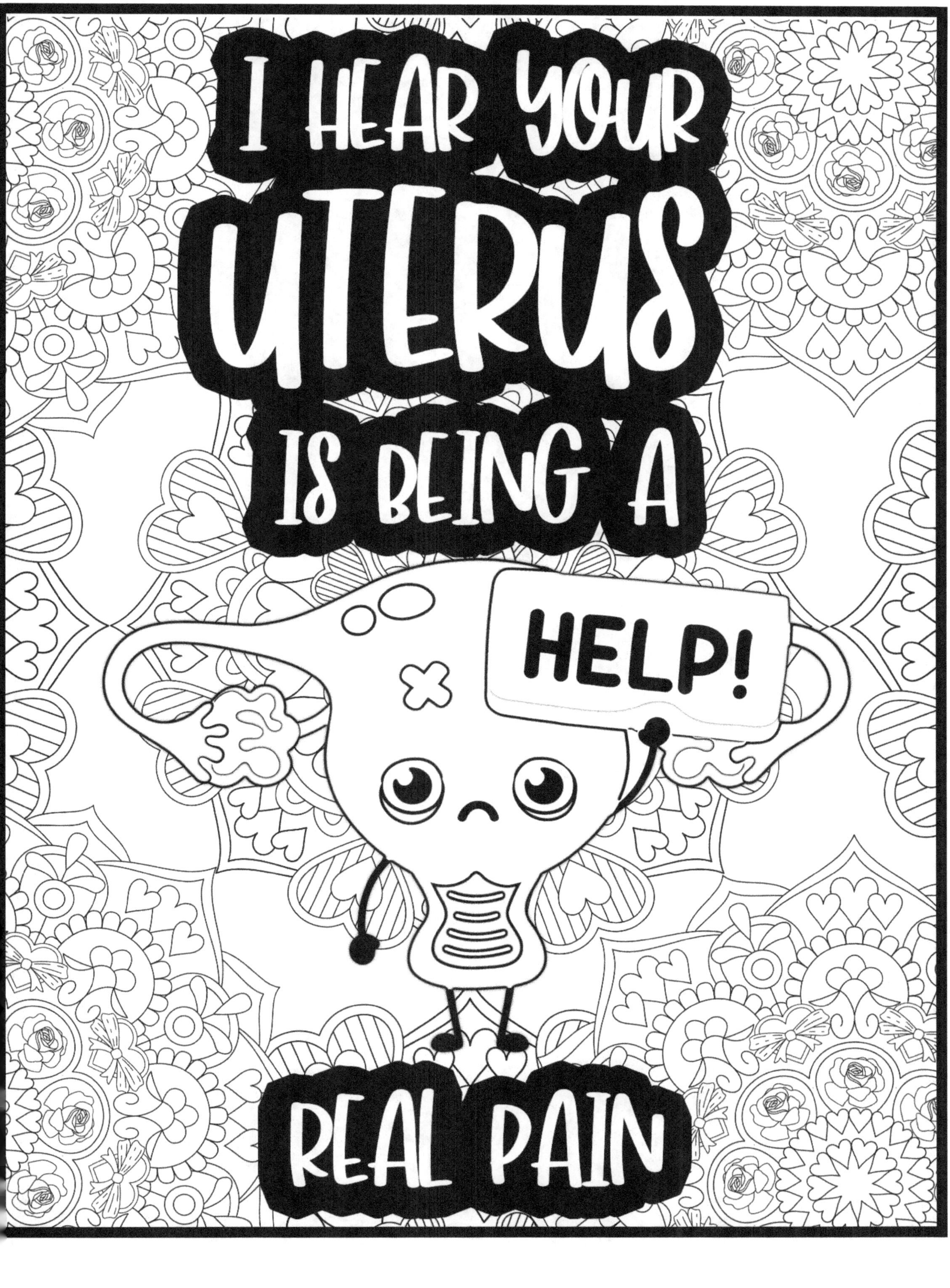

I HEAR YOUR
UTERUS
IS BEING A
HELP!
REAL PAIN

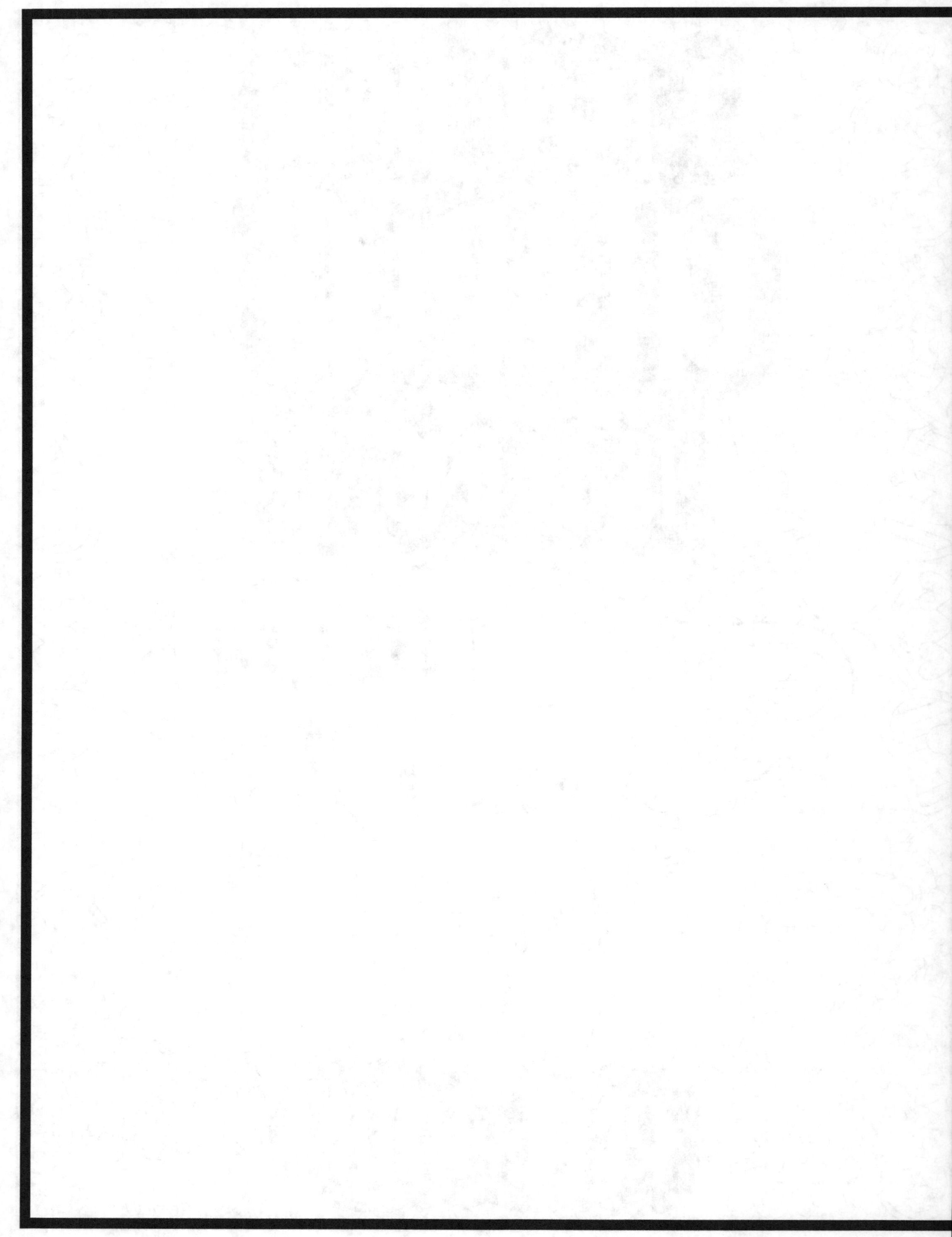

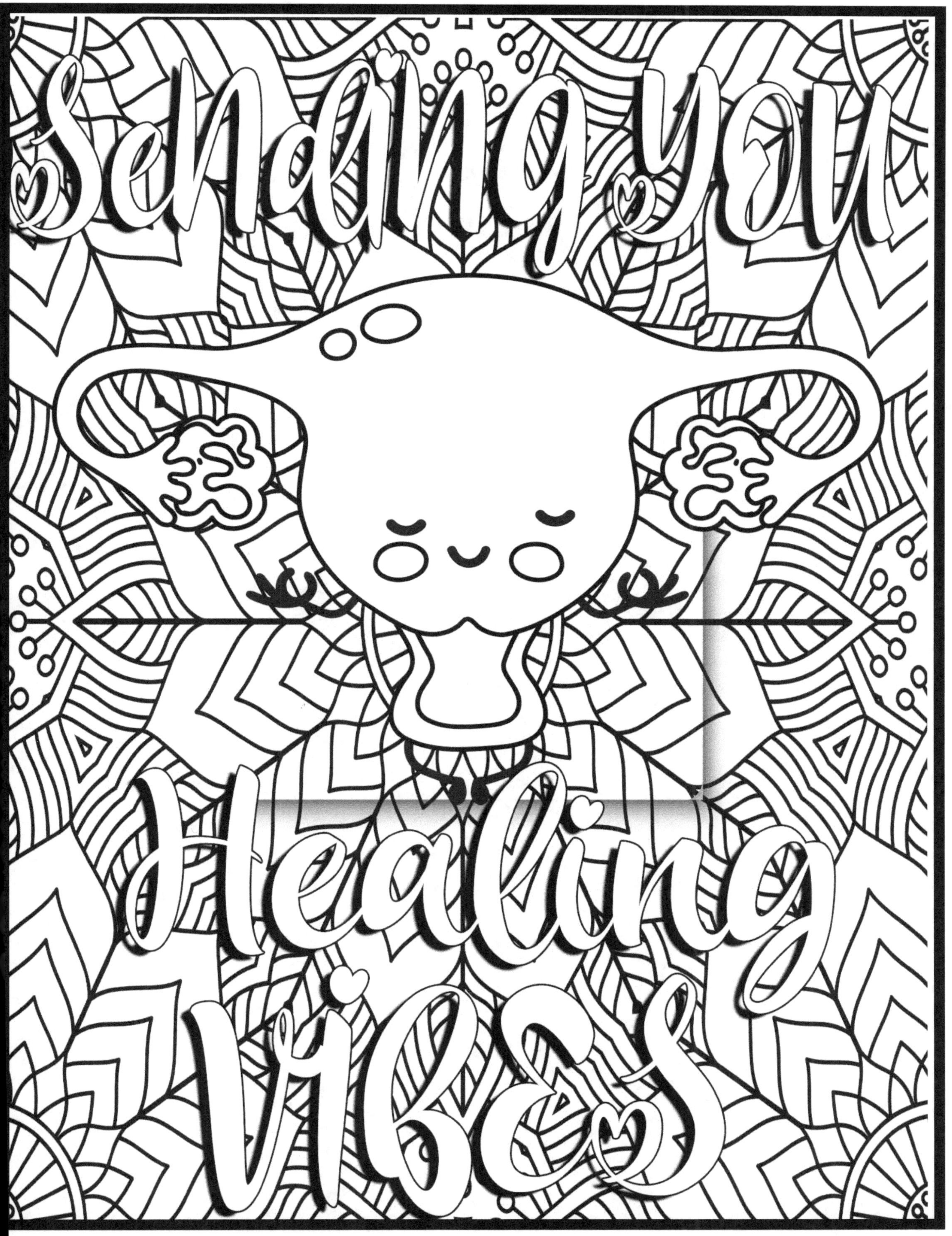
Sending you
Healing Vibes

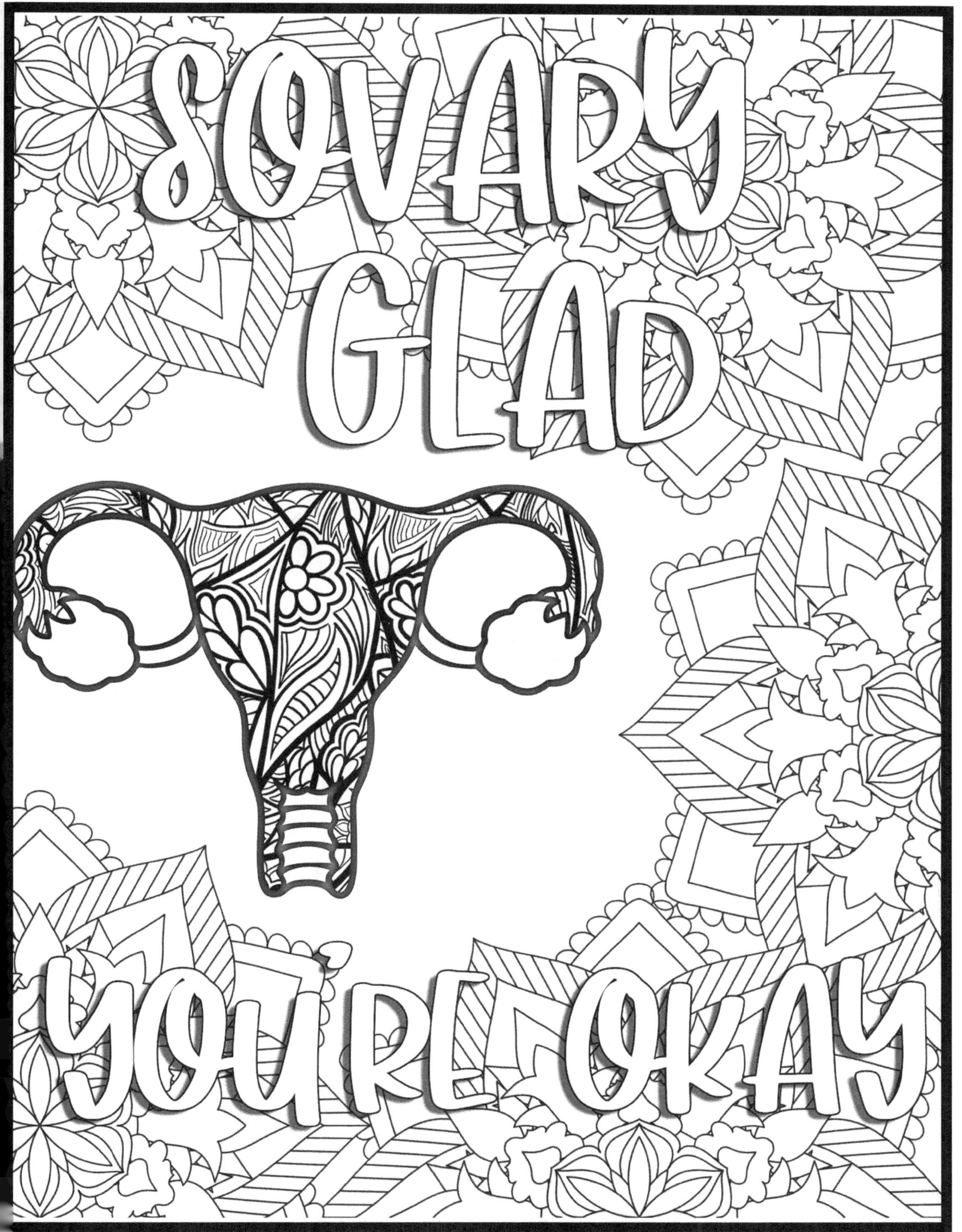

SOVARY
GLAD
YOU'RE OKAY

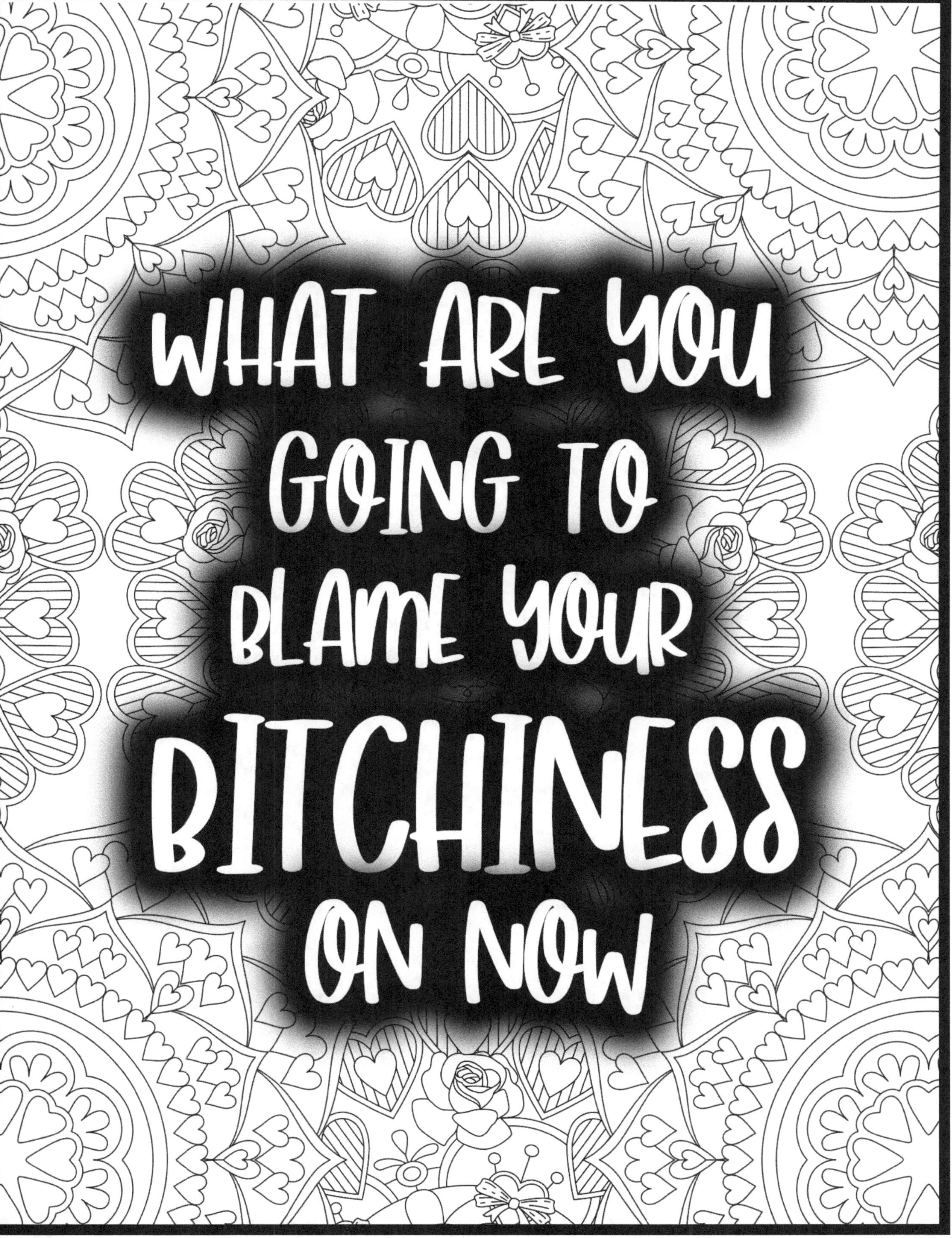

WHAT ARE YOU
GOING TO
BLAME YOUR
BITCHINESS
ON NOW

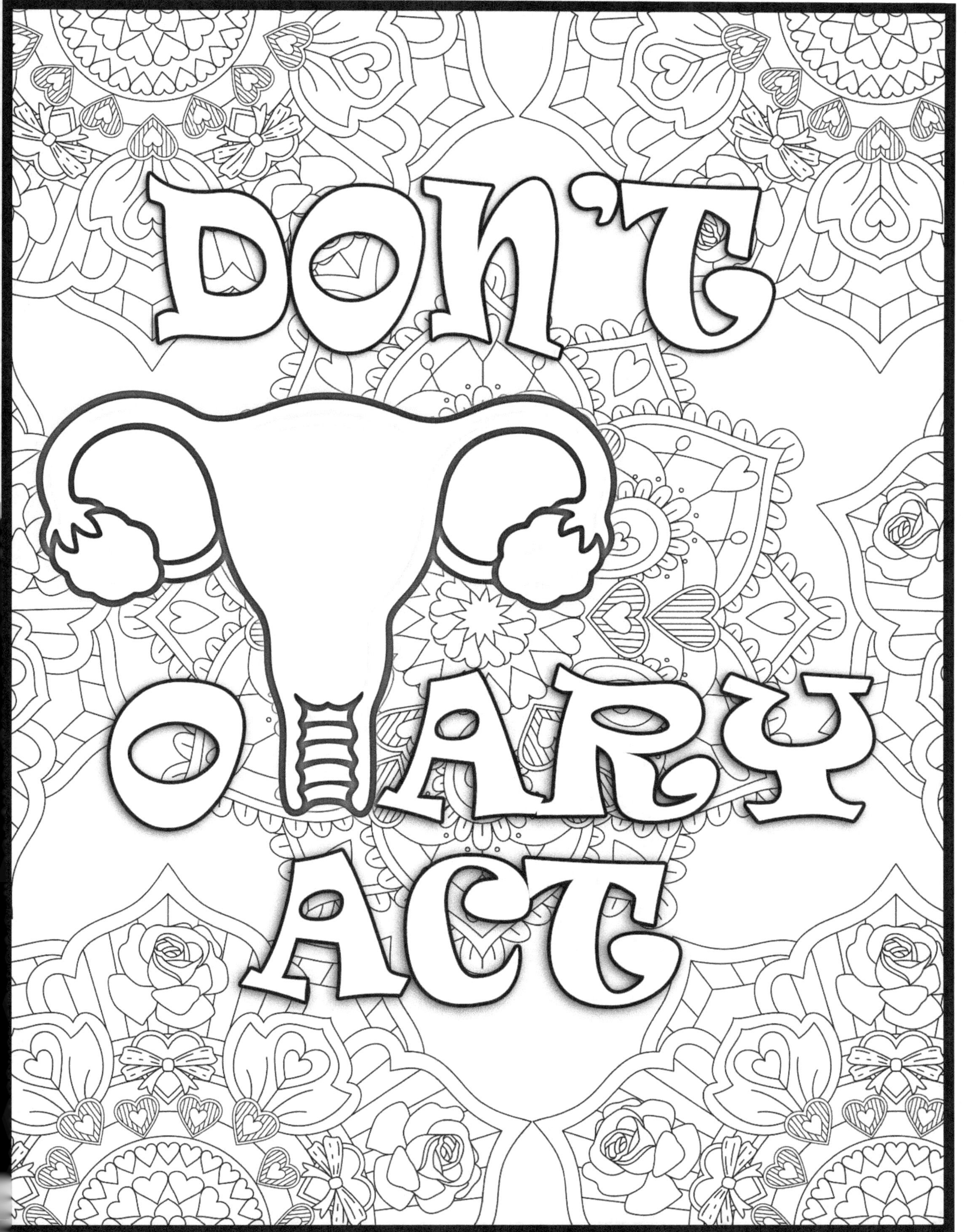

DON'T
OVARY
ACT

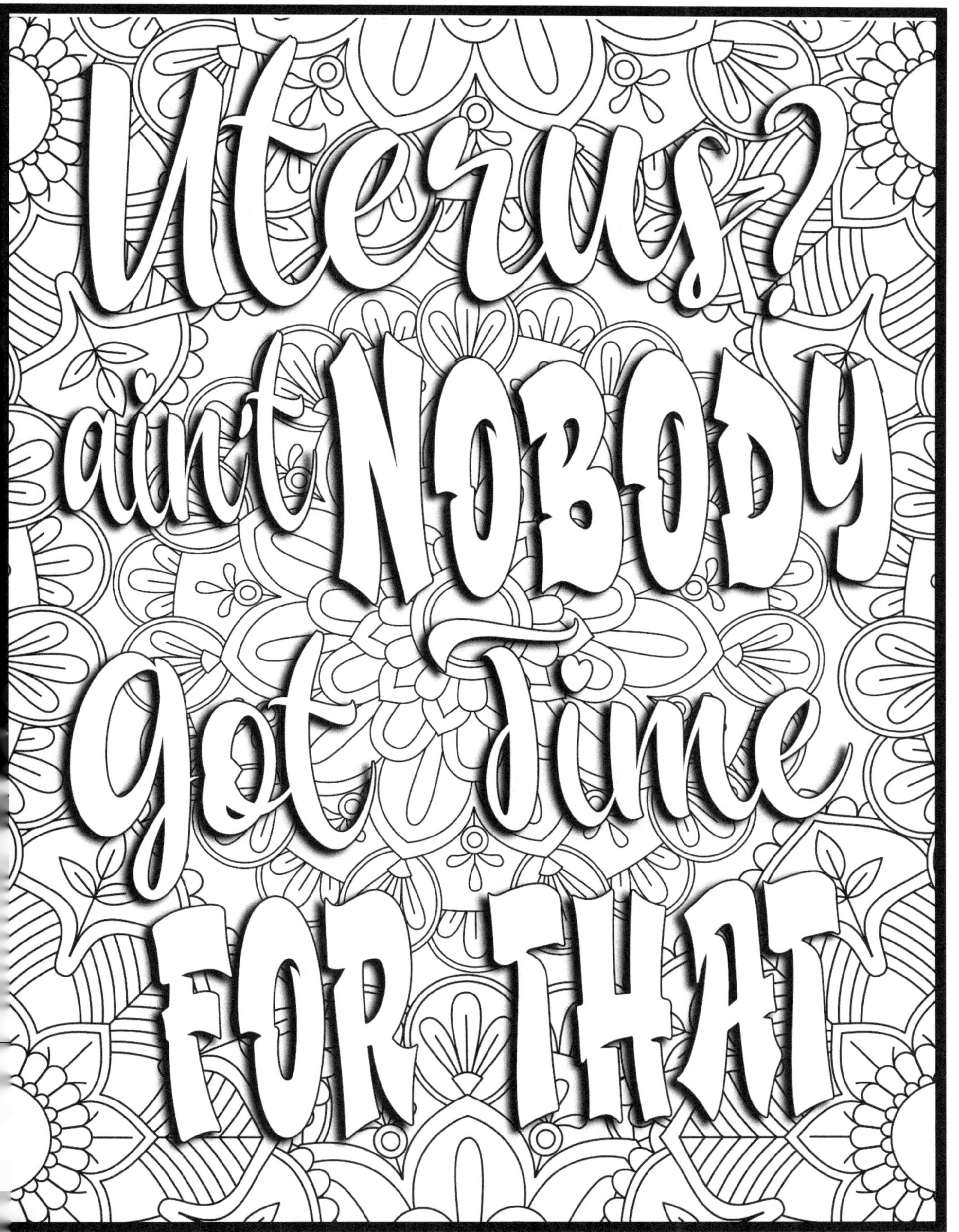

Uterus?
ain't NOBODY
got Time
FOR THAT

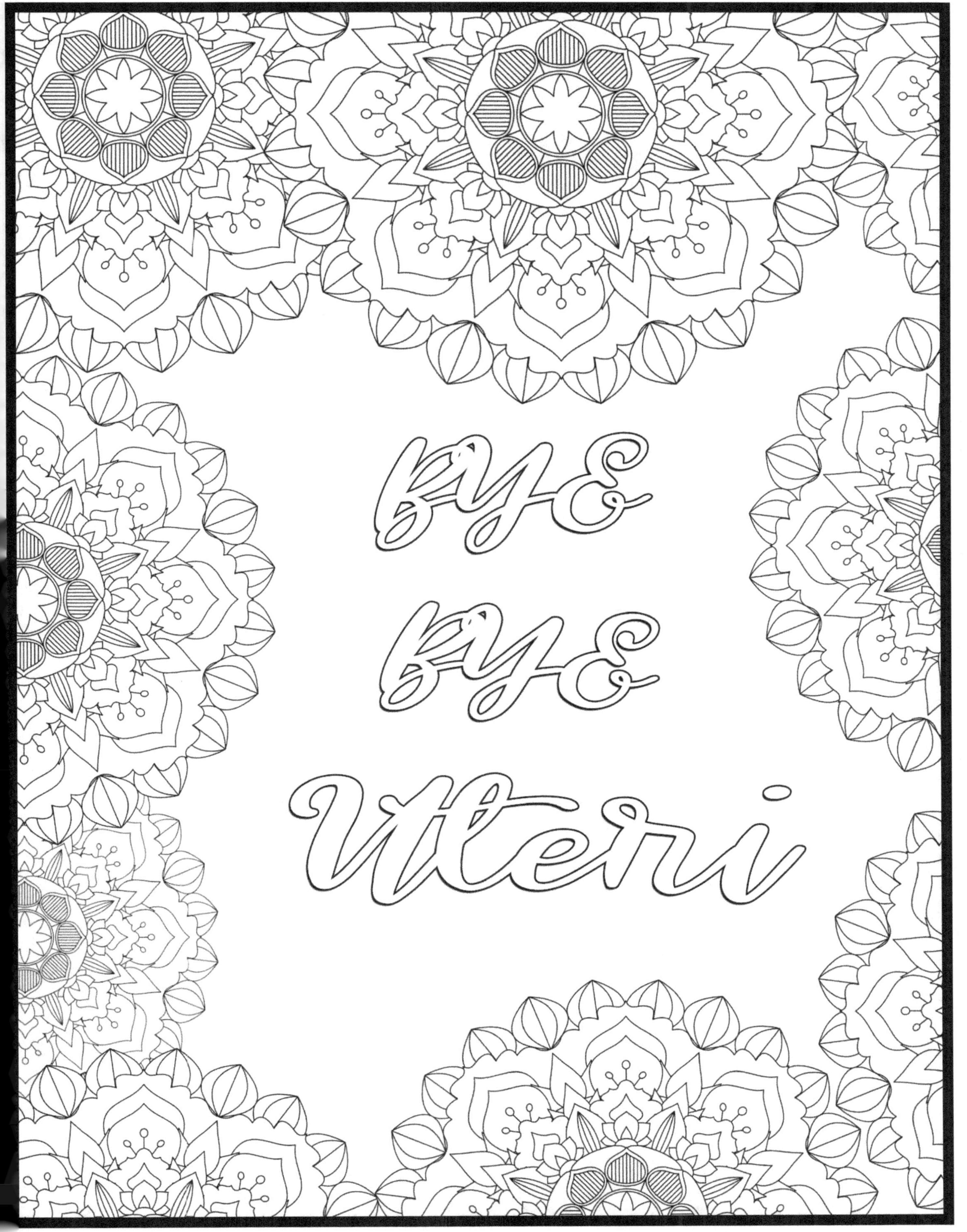

Bye
Bye
Uteri

CAUTION
I MAY
OVARY-ACT
AT ANY TIME

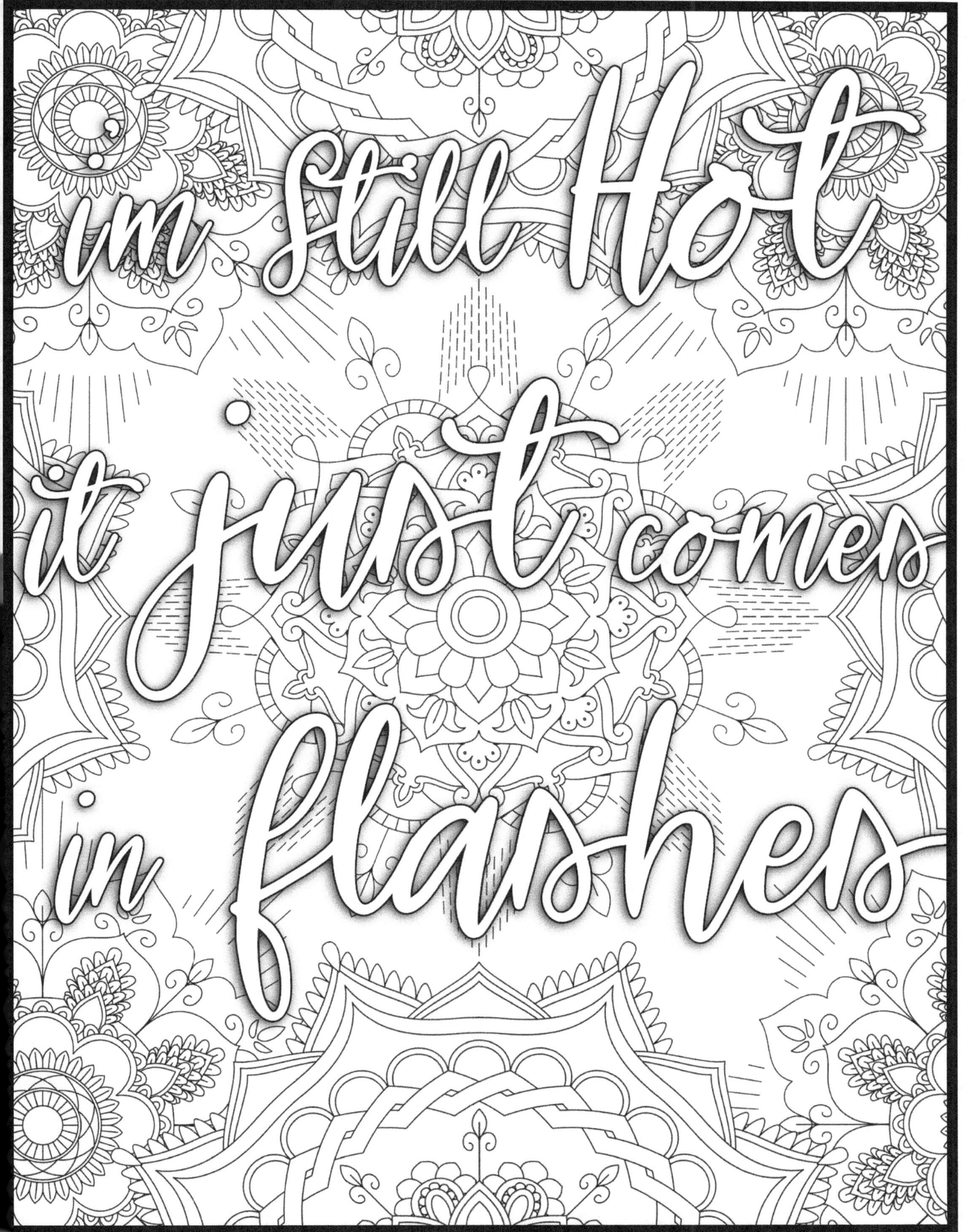

im still Hot
it just comes
in flashes

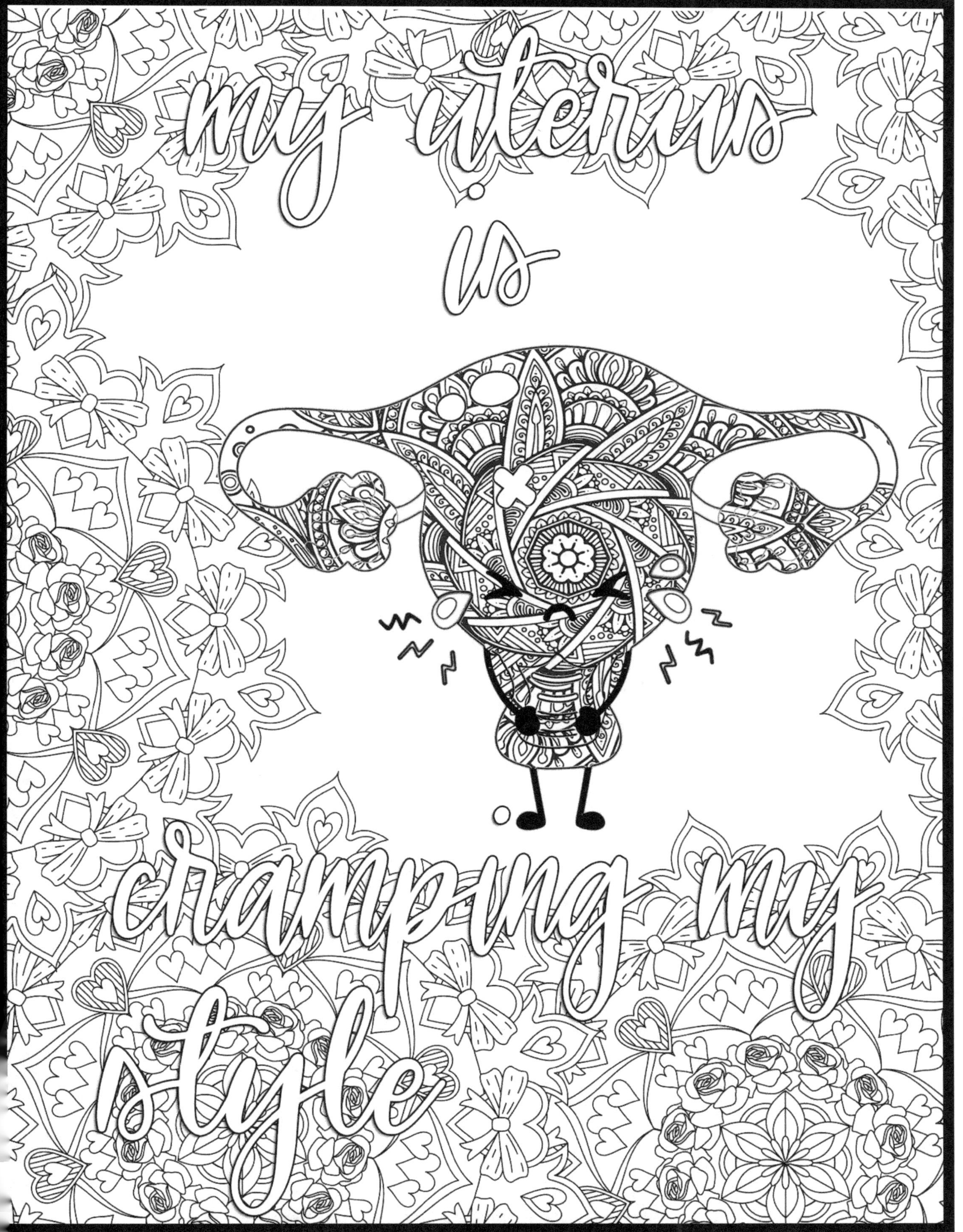

my uterus
is
cramping my
style

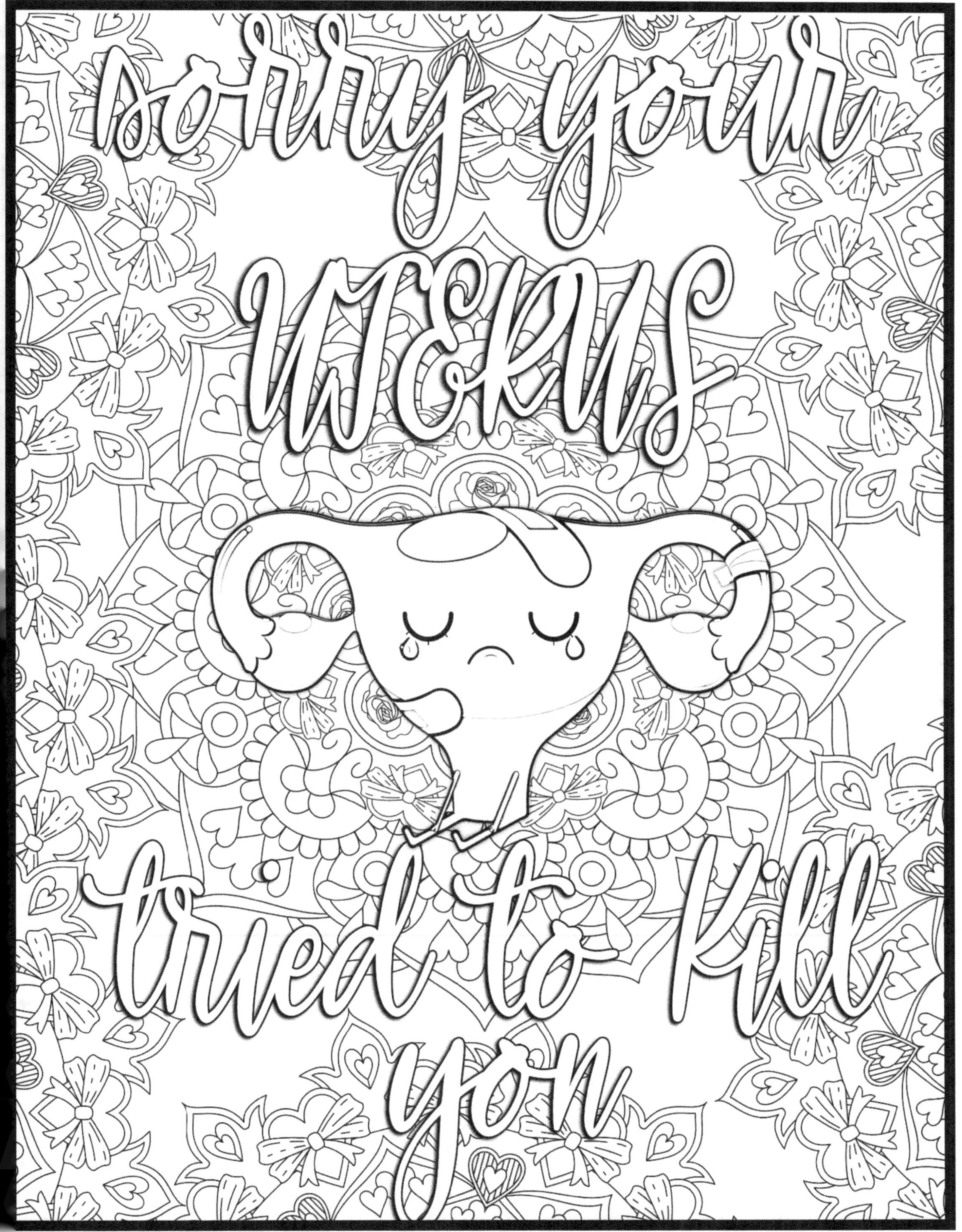

sorry your
WÖMB
tried to kill
you

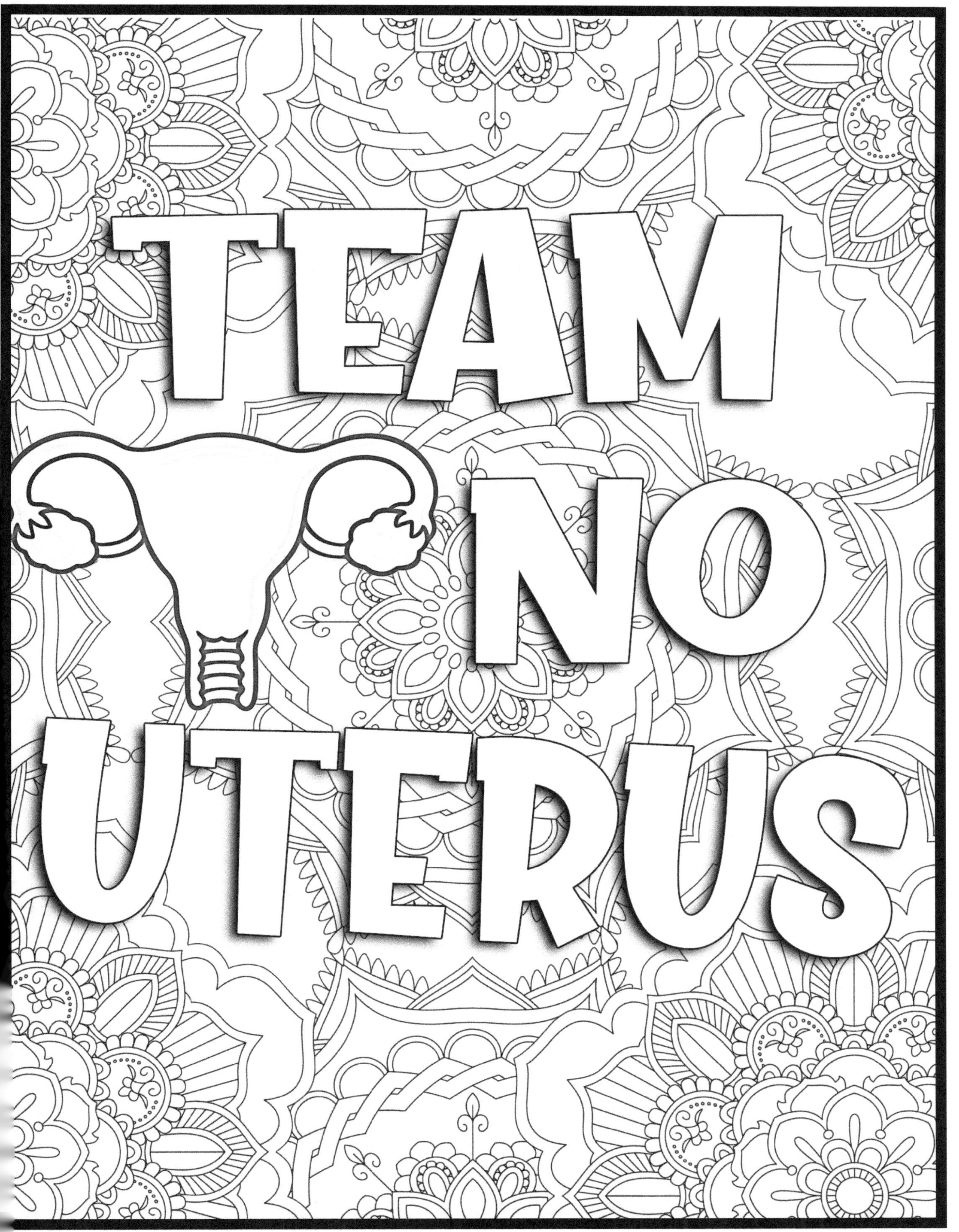

TEAM
NO
UTERUS

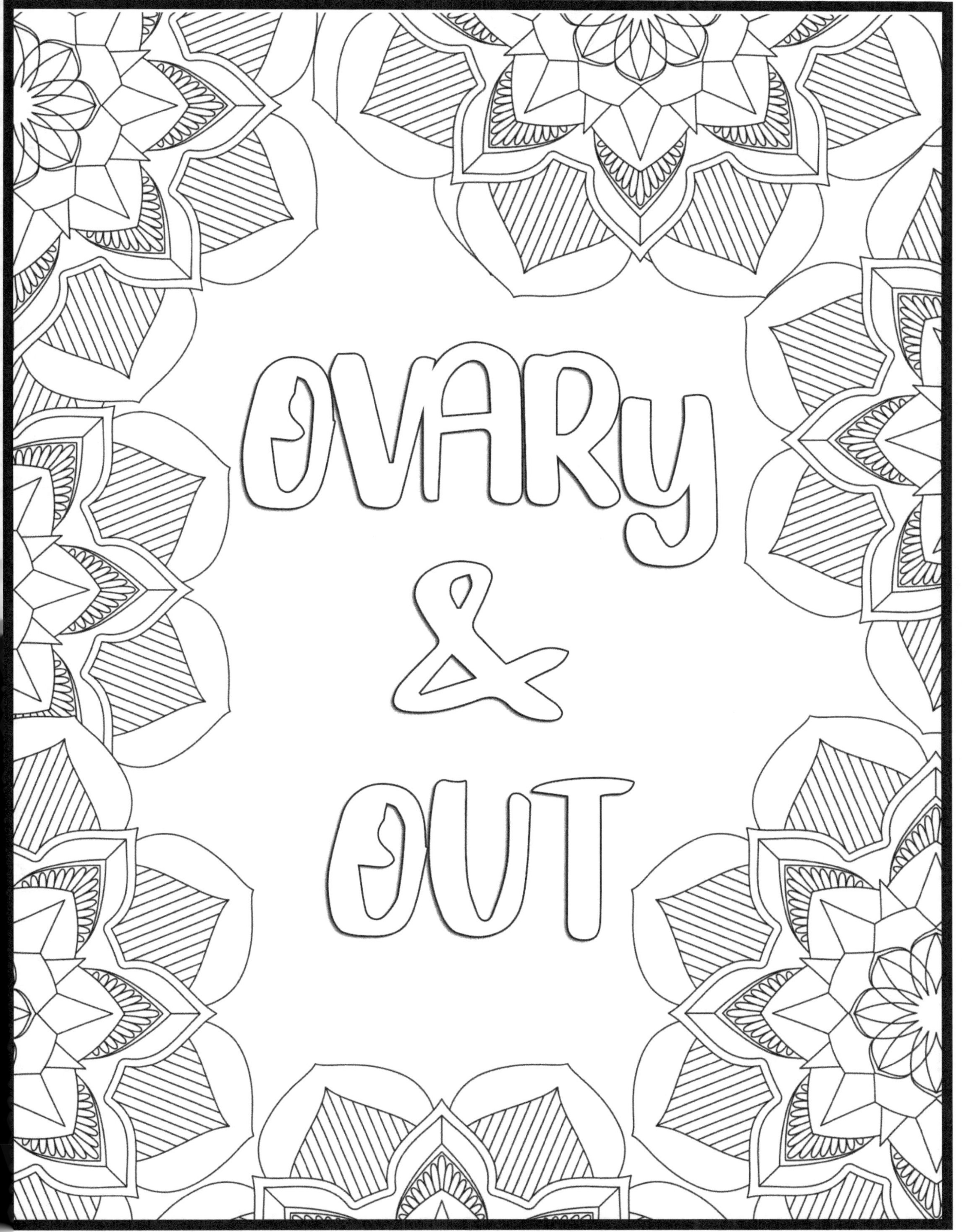

OVARY
&
OUT

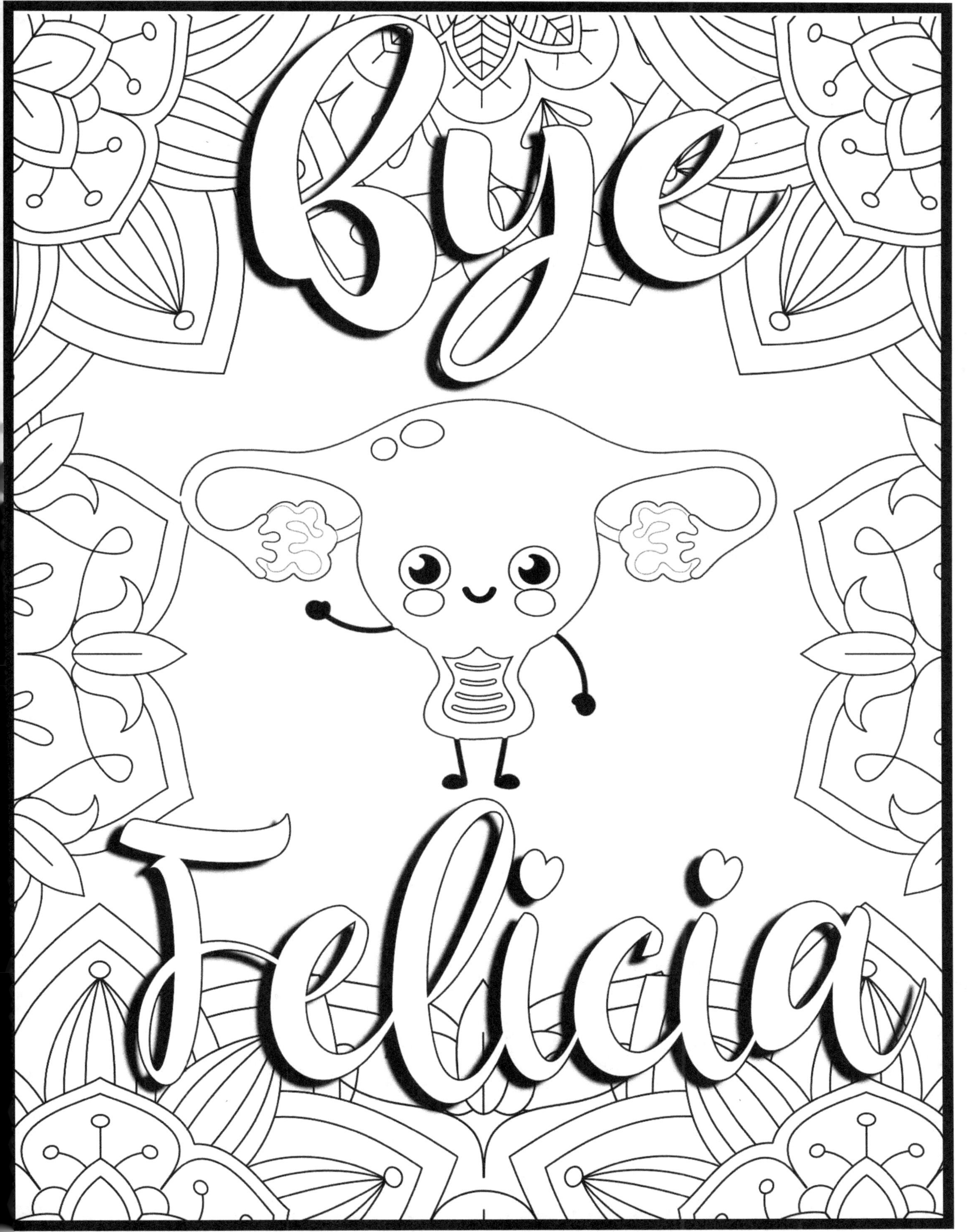

Bye
Felicia

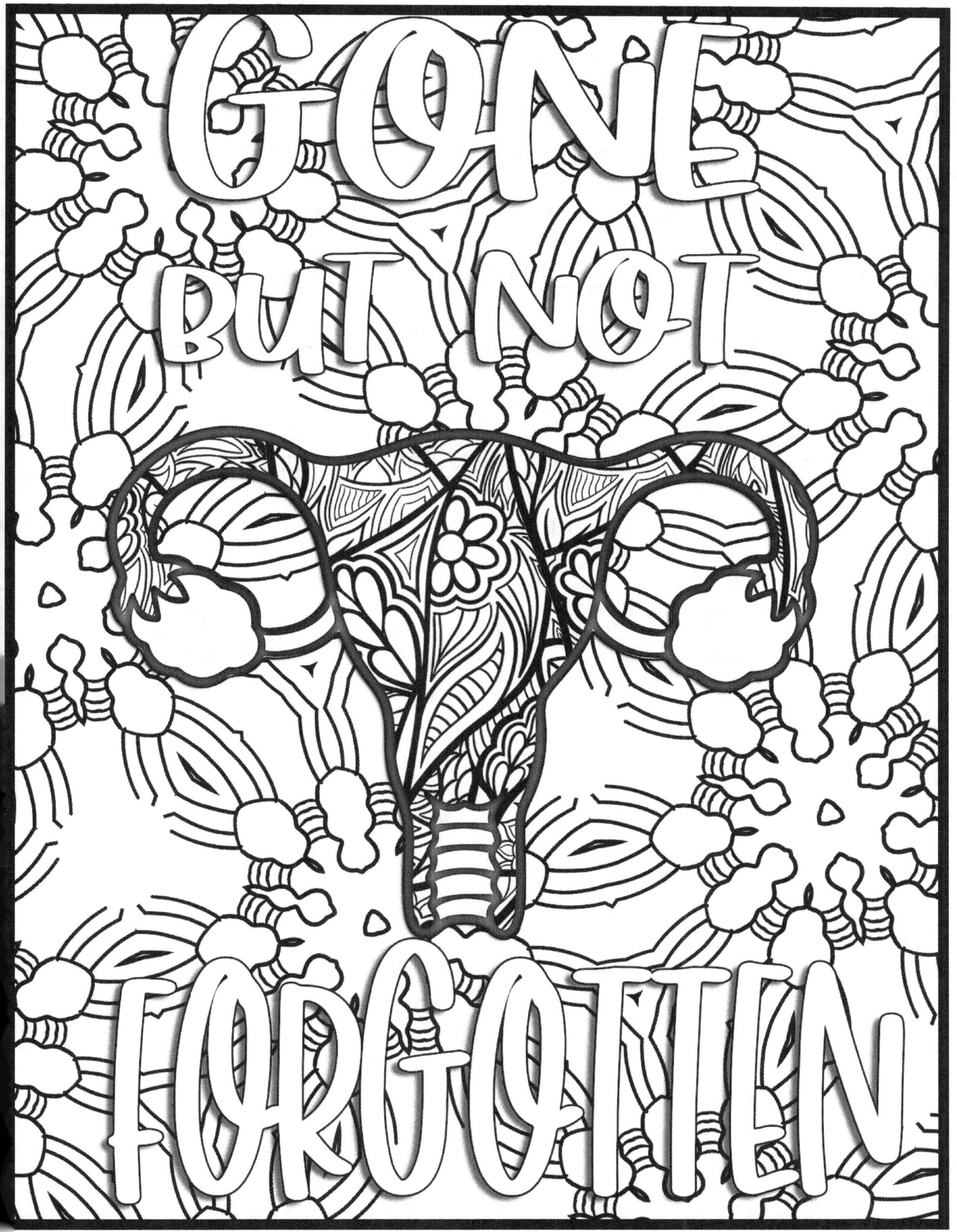

GONE
BUT NOT
FORGOTTEN

Hi, Thank you for purchasing this Hysterectomy Coloring Book. We hope you enjoyed coloring through this stress relieving coloring pages. Let us know what you think about this coloring book by leaving a review. Your opinions or suggestion help us create better products, and also help create a better shopping experience. We value your opinion. Thank you so much for taking time out of your day, we appreciate you!

Best regards